Acupuncture for
WEIGHT LOSS
针炎减肥

Sumiko Knudsen

Ph.D
practioner, DK

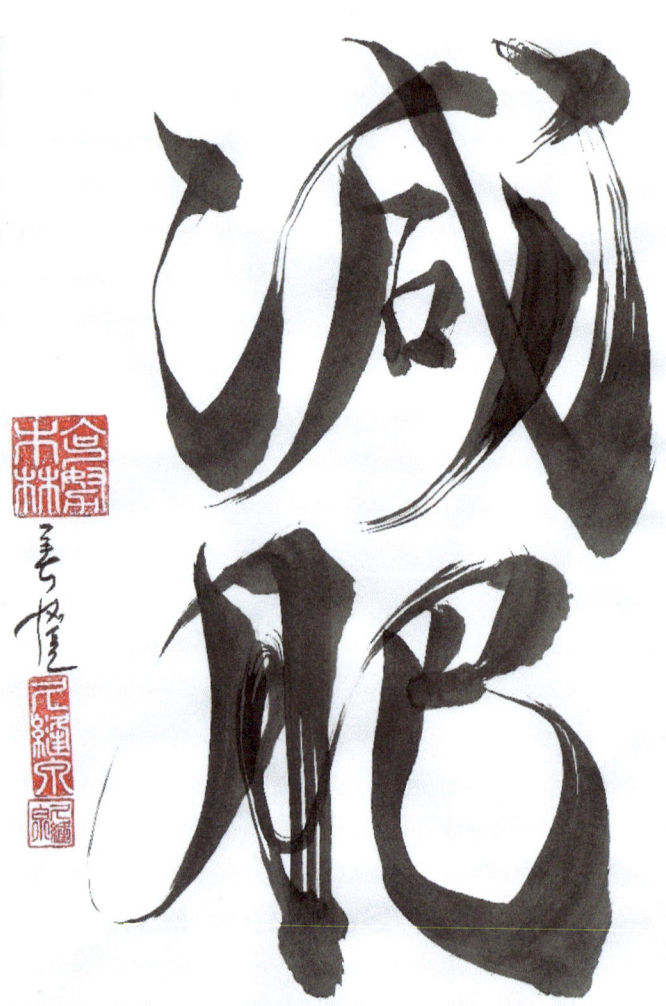

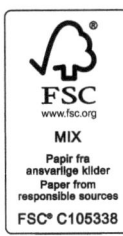

2019 © Sumiko Knudsen
Publisher: BoD – Copenhagen, Denmark
Printing: BoD – Norderstedt, Germany

ISBN: 9788743008699

CONTENTS

INTRODUCTION

Obesity is a serious, wide-spread, stubborn problem. Obesity is a significant risk factor for morbidity and mortality associated with a greater risk for medical conditions including cardiovascular disease, diabetes, hypertension, dyslipidemia, respiratory, osteoarthritis, coronary artery disease, estrogen hormone, gallstone, liver, kidney, depression, pancreatitis, hyperlipidemia and renal etc. Factors of obesity are poor nutrition which is diet and energy metabolism disorder caused by biochemical factor, and among such as fast foods, drugs, food structure, life style, and heredity.

In recent years, treatment of Traditional Chinese Medicine has shown significant results in obesity. This method is nature medicine, non-toxic medicine and has no side-effect in patients. Patients have widely accepted both method of treatment and mechanism of acupuncture in simple obesity, within China and in the world, and it is recognized by WHO.

Acupuncture treatment is non-toxic, no side effects, nature medicine therefore it is recognized, and it has approved by people.

Sumiko Knudsen 克努森澄子

Section 1 Obesity and Weight Loss
肥胖病与减肥

Weight gain and obesity are raising a growing threat to health in countries in the world, and it is a serious issue. Obesity is a chronic disease, prevalent in both developed and developing countries, and affecting even children. Reaching a prevalence of over 396 million worldwide, and it is going to be expected to over 573 million by 2030.

World Health Organization (WHO) on obesity declared definition that chronic diseases associated with cardiovascular, hypertension, certain cancer. Simple obesity classified into adult and children, and childhood obesity is relating heredity. Secondary obesity is, that is, pathological obesity, and it is caused by various diseases such as endocrine, metabolic diseases, and abnormal changes of hypothalamus. Obesity associates with diabetes mellitus and insulin resistance, and obesity results disease of gallbladder, metabolic disturbance, endocrine disturbance, osteoartilitis and gout, pulmonary disease, psychological problem, ovarian function, dyslipidaemia.

In Chinese medicine, it is said that obesity is manifestation of dysfunction of Zang Fu organ and channels, blood, imbalance of Yin and Yang, Yang deficiency and Yin excess, obstruction of dampness and phlegm in internal, and stomach heat. When the failure of Qi to transform the fluid, then it causes retention of dampness to penetrate skin and flesh, and the result will be obesity. Obesity is especially close relation with stomach, spleen, lung, liver and kidney.

In modern medicine, it will be treated by surgical operation, drug, diet and physical exercise. In Chinese medicine treatment is currently by body acupuncture, auricular acupuncture, Catgut embedding, electro acupuncture, combination of body acupuncture and cupping, diet, physical exercise, low-power laser around liver abdominal area.

In clinical research studies, body acupuncture point with efficacy of body acupuncture combined with auricular acupuncture, and observation of patient's undergoing symptoms and signs, body weight, body fat rate, differentiated types and curative effect to the obesity.

1 Definition of Obesity

Obesity is a condition characterized by an abnormal body weight exceeding the normal body weight by more than 20%.

2 Classification of Obesity

- Simple obesity

Simple obesity is that more than 95% of obesity have no obvious reasons.

- Secondary obesity

Secondary obesity is that results from certain disease, which are endocrine and metabolic diseases. Diabetes, insulin resistance, hypothyroidism and pituitary disorders are associated with.

- Classification by body weight

The obesity evaluating indexes include standard body weight and body mass index (BMI).

Standard body weight calculation by height, age and gender.

Standard body weight: (shorter than 155cm) = height-100

Standard body weight: (taller than 155cm) = (height -100) x 0.9

Overweight : 10% of body weight exceeding

Obesity : 20% of body weight exceeding

Mild obesity : 20-30% of body weight exceeding

Moderate obesity : 30-40%

Severe obesity : more than 40%

Section 2 Obesity on Modern Medicine

现代医学对肥胖症认识

2.1 Factor of Obesity

(1) Constitutional

Yellow Emperor recognized that obesity is related with congenital and pointed out when some people are fat and strong, some people are fat and greasy, and some people are constitutionally fat. This is similar to the modern medicine which is obesity is heredity. Such as Qi deficiency of Kidney, and Spleen, which lead to stagnation of Phlegm in the body, and then to be develop to obesity. When Qi deficiency causes to Spleen damage which Spleen is in charge of transportation and transformation of food, and if there is a dysfunction of the Spleen, there will be an accumulation of dampness and phlegm causing to be obesity.

(2) Acquired

(2) -1   Improper Diet

Excessive eating, mainly involving over-eating greasy, sweet, spicy foods which transform into heat and produces fire. Having an irregular diet, f. ex. skipping on one meal a day, and after that consume too much food, and having food late night, thus it gives causing stomach heat to dampness. Spleen is in charge of transportation and transformation. When Spleen has dysfunction, it causes dampness and phlegm to get weight gains. Improper diet is also injuring stomach and spleen, and one eats greasy and rich foods, thus it will be injured stomach and spleen, and especially greasy foods will assemble damp-heat and phlegm.

(2) – 2   Aging and Weakness (Qi deficiency)

After the middle age, women in menopause tend to decline Spleen Qi and fail to transport and transform foods and water, which causes accumulation of dampness and phlegm which leads to obesity. Kidney is the root of the congenital constitution, and when kidney Qi become weak or Qi deficient causes dampness and phlegm and to the end to be obesity.

(2) – 3   Lack of Exercise

Yellow emperor stated that "Long periods of lying down impair Qi and sitting impairs flesh" Qi impairment causes Spleen deficiency. If the Spleen Qi is weak and deficient, it will be failure transportation and transform of food, and it remains dampness and turbid phlegm to be obesity. Lack of physical exercise causes poor circulation in body, and Qi and Blood cannot flow in the body and causes stagnation of Qi and Blood which leads to accumulate of phlegm results in obesity.

(2) – 4   Emotional Disorder

Such as sadness, depression and loneliness which may cause stagnation of Qi, and then develop into an accumulation of phlegm that leads obesity. This type of obesity will be occurred mostly young people and middle-aged woman. If there is emotional disturbance, Qi will be stagnated, and it occurs liver stagnation, and Spleen and Stomach fail for their function.

Clinically, it is the result of multiple compound causes, f.ex. pregnant women or post-partum women, lack of exercise, over-intaking of food. The combination of these and including impeded Qi and disturbance of Qi fails in Sanjiao. It also results deficiency of Qi and Blood and weakness in Spleen and Stomach functions of transportation and transformation after childbirth. The greasy fat will stay in the body, and then it will develop to be obesity.

2.2 Pathogenesis

Simple obesity presents body fat, fatty face, neck, back big buttocks, thigh, legs, and abdominal fat with upper and lower area. Moderate patients show fatigue, aversion to heat, profuse sweating, shortness and rapid of breath, dizziness, and palpitations. Serious patients show shortness of breath, chest distension and not easy to move around. Moderate and serious patients follow hypertension, diabetes mellitus, gallstone, osteoarthritis, visceral (estrogen hormone), vascular (renal), kidney, pancreatitis, respiratory, hyperurimia connect with children, depression, breast cancer, spinal cord injury etc.

(1) Excessive Heat in Stomach and Large Intestine

When there is too much heat in the stomach which will injure the Spleen, and the Spleen will become injured and unable to transport and transformation. It becomes an accumulation of dampness. This is characterized by body-fat and feeling palpation. Manifestation indicates excessive amount of appetite, desire to have cold water, dislike heat, profuse sweating, reddish facial completion, dry stool, constipation, red tongue body, yellow coating, wiry pulse, slippery, rapid. That appears about more than 80% of patients.

(2) Dampness due to Spleen deficiency, accumulating Phlegm

The Spleen is not able to transport and transform resulting in accumulation of dampness which will cause obesity. This is characterized by large fat body mass. Manifestation indicates poor appetites, lassitude, heaviness due to dampness, abdominal distension, loose stool, scanty urine, edema in limbs some cases, tongue body pale, swollen, tender, tongue coating thin, greasy, pulse deep, thready (thin), slippery. Cardiovascular disease,

(3) Qi stagnation of Liver

It manifests heavy body, distention and fullness of hypochondria region, emotional problem, irritability, irregular menstruation, amenorrhea, tongue coating thin, white yellow and wiry thread pulse.

(4) Yang deficiency of Spleen and Kidney

It is characterized by body fat mainly circulated the buttocks and lower limbs, facial puffiness, loose muscle and skin, heavy body, signs of fatigue, lack of strength, aversion to cold, cold limbs, loose stool, abdominal distention, impotence, no interest of sex, sore knees, lumber soreness, tongue coating pale, thin, swollen with teeth mark, greasy, pulse deep, thready, weak, slow.

(5) Yin deficiency of Liver and Kidney

Manifested by heavy body, dizziness (top of head), blurred vision, distending headache, lumber pain, hot sensation, low fever in the afternoon, tongue flat red (tip red), little coating showing heat, dry mouth without moisture, pulse thready, thin, rapid, slightly wiry.

Section 3 Etiology and Pathogenesis
肥胖症病因学研究

3.1 Etiology

(1) Genetic factor

From genetic point of view, obesity may be caused by a single gene or by multiple genes defects. Several genetic studies suggest polymorphisms in several genes. Obesity has strong heritability genetic factors. This has been made clear in several twin and adoptee studies, in which obese individuals who were brought up separately followed the same weight pattern of their biological parents and their identical twins of metabolic rate, spontaneous physical activity etc. Twin studies provide the most impressive clinical evidence that genetic factors play an important role in the etiology of obesity in humans. Stunkard et al. studied identical and nonidentical twins who were brought up together and others who were brought up apart. They found similarity of body weight among identical twins, even if they were brought up apart, and concluded that as much as 70% of the variance of obesity could be attributed to genetic factors. Some study found that children having an obese father and not obese mother significantly increased childhood obesity, but children having obese mother and not obese farther, were not associated with the risk of obesity in childhood. University of Cincinnati published that evidence from a multitude of studies, particularly monozygotic twin studies provide strong support for the impact of genetics of individual differences in body weight and adiposity. In modern science has been the understanding of the intricate molecular pathways dictating energy balance. The genetic and molecular mechanisms govern body weight.

Obesity is not a single disease, and more than 300 different genes and gene markers have been identified that are associated with obesity, thus the genetic influences on body weight.

(1)-1 Single Gene Defects

Single gene defects as models of obesity in animals have been known for many years, and more recently have been described in human. The two most prominent single gene defects that cause obesity in animals and humans include obesity and obesity with diabetes, gene coding for leptin and leptin receptor respectively.

Leptin is made in adipose tissue and suppose to signal the brain regarding insufficiency of food intake and decreasing levels of adipose tissue stores in the body. Leptin is a 16-kdprotein produced generally in white subcutaneous adipose tissue and, to a lesser extent, in the placenta, skeletal muscle, and stomach. (rats) leptin has many functions in carbohydrate, bone and reproductive metabolism that are still being solved. The major role of leptin in body-weight regulation is to signal satiety to the hypothalamus. Thus, reduce dietary intake and fat storage while modulating energy spending and carbohydrate metabolism to prevent further weight gain. Higher circulating leptin levels are associated with a greater risk of congestive heart failure and cardiovascular disease, but leptin does not offer increase prognostic information beyond BMI.

(1)-2

The genetic contribution to obesity is not a single gene defect but is the result of a combination of genetic factors summarizes in the genetics of obesity with leptin and leptin receptor. More than 300 genes are involved in the etiology of obesity, and 24 chromosomes have genes that definitely contribute to obesity. The implications of this number of genes being involved in obesity are that there may be dozens to thousands of different types of obesity.

(2) Nervous, Endocrine and Metabolic factor

Thyroid disease is most often for causing obesity, particularly in puberty. Hypothyroidism produces very rarely significant weight gain and treatment of thyroid deficiency rarely results in weight loss. Hypothyroidism makes it difficult for patients to lose weight while participating in an obesity treatment program, but thyroid hormone replacement, weight loss in response to diet, exercise, and behavior modification such as diet and exercise. Normally thyroid disease is found in obese patients, so it is good to check the serum thyroxin (T4) and TSH before starting a weight-reduction program. Cushing syndrome has result of glucocorticoids is the most common way of endocrine obesity. Obesity with glucocorticoid treatment in the range of 25 to 50kg.

Insulinomas are another cause of endocrine obesity. Pseudohypoparathyroidism, hypothalamic disease and hypogonadism are very rare causes of obesity.

Body adiposity is regulated a long time. Involving insulin and leptin signal to the central nervous system (CNS), especially the hypothalamus of food intake and energy spending. Central nervous system (CNS) regulates system, and to contribute to anabolic and catabolic signaling systems to complete the feedback loop. It indicates shared intracellular signaling from leptin and insulin is provided. The satiety system for meals which consists of neural afferents of the posterior section of the brain from the gastrointestinal tract, and its effectiveness is shown to variety of the strength of insulin and leptin signals.

Stability of body adiposity over long periods marked variation in daily food intake and energy expenditure. Signal generated in body fat acting in the brain to promote energy homeostasis. Variety of circulating nutrients was proposed to function as adiposity signals to the brain. Central nervous system (CNS) is taken up by insulin recognizing serum insulin circulates at concentrations proportionate to body adiposity. That is, insulin provides feedback to the CNS to participate in food intake and body weight regulation. CNS regulates body adiposity. Hormone is secreted from adipocytes stored fat via mechanisms that are ongoing metabolic activity of fat tissue and total body fat content. Leptin showed significantly inhibit food intake and body adiposity in peripherally or centrally. Thus, leptin is like insulin which gives signal to a peripheral to the CNS that participates in the long-term regulation of body weight. Insulin receptors were identified in brain and shown to be concentrated in the hypothalamus and like the peripheral insulin receptor. (53)

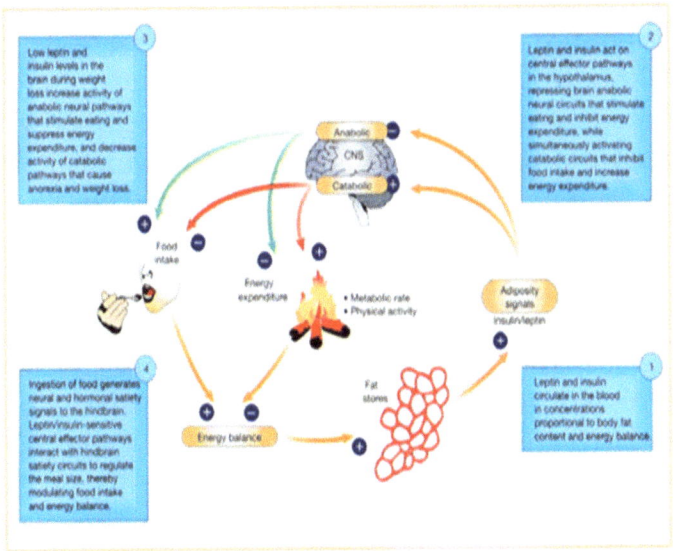

Figure 1 Model showing how a change in body adiposity is coupled to compensatory changes of food intake. Leptin and

insulin are adiposity signals, secreted in proportion to body fat content, which act in the hypothalamus to stimulate catabolic,
while inhibiting anabolic, effector pathways. These pathways have opposing effects on energy balance (the difference
between calories consumed and energy expended) that in turn determines the amount of body fuel stored as fat.
Figure modified from (52).

(3) Psychological factor

The American Psychiatric Association has never regarded overeating or excess weight as a psychiatric disorder, and most studies do not find a clear association between mental health and weight. But some research suggests that depressed persons are more likely to develop the metabolic syndrome that often accompanies excess weight, especially when this weight is concentrated around the waist. People console themselves with comfort food, which is usually high in fat, sugar and calories because they are anxious, lonely, angry or suffering from. There is a characteristic type of depression with symptom of listlessness and overeating, and thus obesity leads to depression and anxiety. National Institute of Health (NIH) edited that obesity increased the risk of onset of depression of older persons. When NIH studied the age 70-79 years old, abdominal obesity predicted onset of depressive symptoms after adjustment for sociodemographic. When BMI and visceral fat were adjusted for each other, only visceral fat was significantly associated with depression onset, and appear mostly in men. Thus, specific mechanisms might relate visceral fat to the onset of depression. Depression is associated with weight gain in about 10 to 20% of cases. Weight gain is particularly common in seasonal depression, which occurs in the winter in northern latitudes. Seasonal affective disorder is associated with weight gain which may be treated by exposure to artificial sunlight. Many patients report that the onset of obesity occurred with some major emotionally stressful event in their lives. Emotional disturbances, such as sadness, depression and loneliness that causes stagnation of Qi, and finally develop into an accumulation of phlegm which leads to obesity. This type of obesity mostly occurs in the young or middle-aged women.

(4) Life style, Diet and Environmental factor

Nowadays many people spend many hours at their desk, television and computer, while devoting only a few hours to physical training or activities. Some studies have shown that watching television for more than 2 hours a day has been linked obesity. Some people live without sidewalk or park and limited to the house and there are nonphysical activities such as not walk to the store or work. Nowadays we can buy many things including foods and fruits through internet, and they send via post or delivery service, so people do not need to go out in supermarket or department store, so in result, it will be lack of physical movement for people. It was found by researcher that environmental changes such as moving to a new country f. ex. Asian country to Europe, it can be led to different eating habits and daily foods which in turn leads to weight gain. Some people whom their life style is very limited such as eating fast food, sugared beverage intake, and if it continues to intake of excessive fatty foods a long time, it may cause dysfunction of Spleen Qi which leads to stagnation of phlegm in the body and finally leads to obesity. For school children, it is an important to have nutrition of food from school lunch program with low fat calories and provides physical activity into regular routines daily behaviors. As school lunch, it is necessary to promote healthier choices including at least 5 different of fruits and vegetables a day, reasonable portion sizes of food and beverage for decreasing excessive calorie consumption. Children living in European countries, obesity was independently associated with use of electronic games and television and it was negatively associated with physical activity. Children in European countries would like to avoid "toxic environment" leading to the childhood obesity epidemic which already experienced in USA. (110)

Macronutrient content of the diet which is carbohydrate, protein and fat, energy density, sugar-sweetened in beverages, and portion size has been involved obesity trend. The studies in University of Cincinnati, USA showed the evidence that monounsaturated fats which diet is most popular in the Mediterranean region in Europe emphasizes the effects of the consumption of vegetables, fruits, whole grains, legumes, nuts, olive oil and canola oil and limit the intake of saturated fats from meat poultry, and dairy products. Results showed that high monounsaturated fats diets may improve weight, blood pressure, plasma lipids, and insulin sensitivity and lower fat diets. Lower carbohydrate, higher protein diets are associated with superior benefits for weight loss. A low-calorie diet provides about 1000 to 1500 Kcal per day and this depends on body weight. Most obesity guidelines recommend decrease fat intake to less than 30% of total calorie intake.

Diet and physical activity contribute to energy balance and weight control. Multi-strategy interventions that include educational, behavioral, f. ex. problem solving, goal setting, and self-monitoring and environmental approaches have been effective in promoting healthy lifestyle habits in the short-term. So, it is imperative that well-designed, large-scale trials be conducted to establish the long-term efficacy of specific strategies and delivery methods for the prevention and control of obesity in home, school, workplace, and healthcare settings. The environment includes many factors that can lead to weight gain such as work, stress, and other lifestyles habits.

There are many environmental factors that appear to be necessary for the expression of obesity. Obesity is the interaction of the environment and genetic tendency to accumulate excess adipose tissue. Regulation of energy balance is compound and influenced by numerous genetic and environmental factors. Both the genetic factor and the environmental factor present for obesity to occur.

3.2 Pathogenesis
3.2.1 Risk of Disease Associated with Obesity

Obesity causes by an extreme accumulation of body fat tissue mass and escalates of health problem. It is associated with increased fat cell size and number, and it usually followed by serious health consequences if not controlled. It causes both independently and in association with other diseases. Body weight and storage of energy as triglyceride in adipose tissue are determined by the interaction between genetic, metabolic associated with several specific biochemical, environmental, and psychological factors. These influences act eventually act by changing the balance between energy intaking and spending. Obesity has increased and become global problem with a number of pathological disorders, and obesity has closely connected with disease like hypertension, diabetes mellitus type 2, cardiovascular disease, cancer, stroke, osteo-arthritis, dyslipidemia, gallstones, respiratory system, Liver, Kidney, depression and sleep-apnoea. Obesity brings into many diseases and complications and accelerates ageing and even to increase mortality. An extensive number of epidemiological studies have established a significant increase in cardiovascular and non-cardiovascular mortality associated obesity. (89)

3.2.2 Obesity associated disease

(1) Diabetes

The long-term risk of type 2 diabetes increases significantly with increasing weight. Several studies have an evidence that weight loss is associated with a significant reduction in the risk of type 2 diabetes which associated with obesity, and weight loss has improved diabetes control. (89) Overweight people have a three times greater risk of becoming diabetic. The increase in fat will change endocrine function. It causes an increase in glucose and resistance to insulin resulting in type 2 diabetes.

(2) Cardiovascular Disease

Obesity is an independent risk factor for Cardiovascular including angina pectoris, myocardial, congestive heart failure, stroke, and hypertension. Results from the Framingham Heart Study showed that obesity increases the risk of atrial fibrillation. Hypertension is a risk factor for cardiovascular and is related to obesity. Women's Health Study found a significant association between obesity. (89)

Cardiovascular disease is one of the major diseases associated with obesity. The excess fat in the body can put excess stress on the heart. The heart must pump more blood causing it to become enlarged resulting in heart failure.

(3) Metabolic Syndrome

Metabolic syndrome is associated with cardiovascular risk factors, and includes abdominal obesity combined with elevated blood pressure, fasting plasma glucose, and triglycerides, and reduced high-density lipoprotein cholesterol levels. Metabolic syndrome is associated with an increased risk of cardiovascular mortality. Abdominal obesity is strongly associated with the risk of diabetes.

(4) Cancer

There is a significant association between obesity and cancer. American Cancer Prevention Study II who were free from cancer in 1982 and followed up to 16 years. Among those with BMI $\geq 40kg/m2$, mortality from all causes of cancer was 52% higher in men and 62% higher in women compared with those with normal BMI. BMI is significantly associated with higher rate of death due to cancer of esophagus, colon, rectum, liver, gallbladder, pancreas, kidney, lymphoma, and multiple myeloma.

It is especially in women that renal cell carcinoma associated with increased BMI, but no significant increase was observed for men by European Prospective Investigation into Cancer and Nutrition study.

(5) Arthritis

Obesity is strongly associated with an increased risk of osteoarthritis of the knee and a moderate association with osteoarthritis of the hip. Osteoarthritis impacts people's lifestyle and function, and it is important to have weight loss. Weight loss has been shown to significantly improve signs and symptoms of osteoarthritis and improve disability and function in obese people.

(6) Gallbladder Disease

The significant connection with obesity and Gallbladder disease among women were by an epidemiologic study at National Health Service in England and Scotland. Women with higher BMI were more gallbladder disease. Gallbladder disease was attributed to obesity.

(7) Acute Pancreatitis

Acute pancreatitis is closely associated with obesity and it will be severity and mortality. Obesity (BMI ≥ 30kg/m2) was identified as a risk factor for the development of local complications in acute pancreatitis and associated with increased mortality.

(8) Liver

Nonalcoholic fatty liver disease is associated with obesity. National Health Survey proved the prevalence of nonalcoholic fatty liver disease was 30% and this was more common in men (38%) than in women (21%), and obesity (BMI>30kg/m2 was independently associated with this disease.

(9) Pulmonary Complications

Obstructive sleep apnea is characterized by upper airway obstruction that occurs as repetitive episodes during sleep. Obstructive sleep apnea is loud snoring, fragmented sleep, repetitive hypoxemia, hypercapnia, daytime sleepiness etc. among middle-aged women and men. Obesity is the most risk factor for the development of obstructive sleep apnea, and 60% to 90% of adults are overweight. Obesity can also affect the lung causing obstruction and difficulties in breathing leading to pulmonary complications.

(10) Depression

The National Epidemiologic Survey evaluated the relationship between BMI and psychiatric disorders, and among participants, BMI was significantly associated with mood, anxiety, and personality disorders.

Research has shown that job related stress can contribute to obesity and overweight.

3.2.3 Treatment of Obesity by Western treatment

The imbalance between energy input and output leads to excess accumulation of fat in the body. Eating habits have changed and it has been increased of calorie intake and not enough physical activities to burn the calories. Weight loss programs ranges from individual planned exercise and diet planning to medical interventions such as surgery and weight loss medications. In order to be managing weight loss to be success, it is most important and necessary to change lifestyle which behavioral changes including dietary ways and physical exercise is one of the key factors for treatment. In order to spend energy, it is necessary to do exercise.

In western treatment of obesity is mainly to eat few calories and to physical excise. If it is extreme case, it could be surgery and medications for weight loss, and besides it is going to be popular alternative medicine.

(1) Diet Therapy

According the recommendation of American College of Sports Medicine, the spending calorie in adults will be 300 to 500 kcal per exercise session or 1,000 to 2,000 kcal per week, and weight loss program should start with losing 10 percent of weight from baseline within six months. The diet should be low in fat and high in fibre, and suitable balance carbohydrate, protein and fat for intaking of the right amount of nutrients, such as vitamins. Obesity management guidelines of the National Heart, Lung, and Blood Institute recommends the low carbohydrate diet with 30g per day or less, and vegetables and fruits with high ratios of fiber to carbohydrate. Group studied for 6 months for weight loss both low carbohydrate diet and low-fat diet.

The low carbohydrate diet was associated with greater decreases in serum triglycerides and greater increases in HDL cholesterol than was the conventional diet.

Mediterranean style diet which food rich in mono and polyunsaturated fat, fiber and low ratio of omega-6 to omega 3 fatty acids are also associated with weight loss. Studies provide evidence for the influence of portion size on energy intake at a single meal, the impact on body weight may be minimized if persons compensate by consuming less energy at the next meal. After examined, it showed the effect of larger portions of all foods over 2 days period. Results showed a 26% increase in energy intake on both days of feeling fuller.

(2) Physical Excise Therapy

Walking can be safely performed and easily incorporated into daily life. Excising could be aerobic including body toning, Zumba dancing, cycling, swimming, jogging, climbing stairs, walking greater distances, gardening, housework, and at least 30 minutes of moderate intensity physical activities.

Exercise is the best predictor of preventing recurrent weight gain. It is more effective to get guidelines for activity prescription for aerobic activity or fitness training for daily lifestyle activities. Main components of the exercise prescription are provided warm-up and cool-down periods are necessary. Strength training is effective for obesity treatment using hand weight, body bar, even carrying grocery bags from daily living. Physical activity should be initiated at a slow pace for short periods of time and gradually increased in intensity and time.

(3) Drug therapy
may be helpful part of treatment for overweight and obesity along with diet, physical exercise, and behavior changes. Most people regain their weight when they have stopped using drugs. People should know and understand that evaluation of drug for risks and benefits before making decision. Drug therapy can be useful with BMI greater than 30 kg/m2. It should be used in combination with an instructed diet and an exercise program to achieve the greatest and longest lasting results. The effect of weight loss obtained through the use of drug therapy on overall morbidity and mortality has not been established.

Medication in main role for obesity mainly falls into appetite suppressant, metabolic stimulants, digestion and absorption inhibitors, insulin sensitizers, and fat and fat cell inhibitors;

(1) Appetite Suppressant

It referred to anorectic drugs which are used adjuncts to behavioral therapy in weight reduction program. The two classes of anorectic drugs are noradrenergic and the serotonergic agents. Noradrenergic drugs affect weight loss through action in the appetite center. Phenylpropanolamine (Dexatrim), a sympathomimetic drug and synthetic derivative of ephedrine, is as an over the counter appetite suppressant and decongestant and have a greater weight loss. Side effects are causing nervousness, insomnia, dizziness, palpitations and headaches. This drug is treated also as patients have high blood pressure, depression or anxiety disorder, or if they have diabetes, heart disease or thyroid disease.

Drug of Phentermine is to regulate noradrenergic neurotransmission to decrease appetite and used for as a single weight loss agent.

(2) Metabolic Stimulants

The combination of Ephedrine and caffeine possesses anorectic and thermogenic properties. Ephedrine increases the release of Norepinephrine which regulates food intake and acts as a sympathomimetic agent to stimulate heart rate and blood pressure and increase themogenesis. Caffeine, an adenosine antagonist, reduces the breakdown of Norepinephrine within the synaptic junction. Side effect of using combination of Norepinephrine and caffeine causes tremor, insomnia and dizziness.

Selective beta-adrenergic agonists are to increase the rate of metabolism and cause weight loss by decreasing the body lipid. Mutation in the gene coding for the beta-Adrenergic receptor is associated with weight gain, abdominal obesity and insulin resistance.

(3) Digestion and Absorption Inhibitors

It is to use digestive inhibitors that interfere with the breakdown, digestion and absorption of dietary fat in the gastrointestinal tract, such as gastric and pancreatic lipases aid in the digestion of dietary triglycerides by forming them into free fatty acids that are absorbed at the border of the small intestine.

Inhibition of these enzymes leads to inhibition of the digestion of dietary triglycerides and decreased cholesterol absorption, and may decrease absorption of lipid soluble vitamin A, D, E and K. Gastrointestinal side effects occurred in as many as 40 percent of patients and resulted in discontinuation of use in about 10 percent of patients. (122) Gastrointestinal side effects are accumulation of gas in the stomach, oily stool, feces incontinence and abdominal pain. Orlistat is currently the only available drug that alters fat digestion. It is inhibitor of pancreatic lipases, and this does the absorption of about 30 percent of dietary fat. Orlistat is indicated for use in patients with BMI of at least 30 kg/m2 or in patients with hypertension, diabetes or dyslipidemia who have BMI of greater than 27 kg/m2. It demonstrated that 55% of patients treated with Orlistat at the recommended dose of 120 mg and lost more than 5% of their body weight. 25% of patients took Orlistat and lost 10% of their body weight. But Orlistat showed down the rate of weight regain in the second year of treatment.

(4) Insulin Sensitizers

Such as Sibutramine agent which is used for diabetes, but also used for patients whom have BMI over 30kg/m2. Obesity is associated with diabetes type 2, and alteration of in the gene coding for the beta-adrenergic receptor is associated with weight gain, abdominal obesity and insulin resistance. In diabetic patients, Sibutramine resulted in significantly lost weight.

(5) Fat Inhibitors

This is to decrease caloric value from fat while maintaining the creaminess and richness derived from fat. The most recent fat-based substitute is Olestra which contains zero kcal per g. Olestra is a sucrose polyester, and for using as a food additive in prepackaged snacks such as potato, corn and tortilla chips, and crackers to replace 100 percent of the fat. As a sucrose polyester with six to eight fatty acid side chains, it is too large to be hydrolyzed by digestive enzymes, therefore, it is not absorbed and has no caloric value. A 28g serving of potato chips fried in fat contains 10g of fat and 150 calories, while a similar serving of Olestra potato chips contains no fat and only 70 calories. 4 weeks study has shown that 4 kg weight loss when Olesta was substituted for dietary fat in a hypocaloric diet. Olestra may be effective improvement weight loss when used in a calorie restricted diet. Side-effect of Olesta is to cause gastrointestinal, such as bloating, flatulence, diarrhea, loose stools and anal leakage. Olesta may inhibit the absorption of fat-soluble vitamin A, D, E and K and carotenoids. The absorption of fat-soluble vitamins from the digestive tract can only be affected by the presence of Olestra if the both foods are eaten at the same time.

(4) Surgical Therapy

Surgical therapy for obesity may be considered if;

•People have with body mass index (BMI) of 40 or higher.

•BMI of 35 to 39.9, and have a serious weight related health problem, such as diabetes or high blood pressure.

•People committed to have the lifestyle changes that are necessary for surgery to work.

Surgical therapy for weight loss is offering the chance of losing the most weight, but it can be risks. This surgery limits the amount of food to eat and decreases absorption of food and calories. Surgery can help about 50 percent of excess body weight, but it has no guarantee to lose all of excess weight or keeping it off long term.

Weight loss for obesity surgeries include:

1)Gastric bypass surgery

The small intestine is operated a short distance below the main stomach and connected to the new pouch which created small pouch at the top of stomach, and then food and liquid flow directly from the pouch into this part of the intestine, bypassing stomach.

2)Laparoscopic adjustable gastric banding (LAGB)

It creates a small channel between the two pouches. This will not work without changes in people's behavior, and the result is usually not as good. The Lap Band gastric banding device has not been approved people who have BMI of 30 to 34 and if people have an additional health condition related to their obesity.

3)Gastric sleeve

Part of the stomach is removed and creating a smaller reservoir for food. This procedure is still ongoing studies for evaluating.

4)Biliopancreatic diversion with duodenal switch

Most of stomach is removed by this procedure. It will be big risk for malnutrition and vitamin deficiencies, and it is necessary to take close medical monitoring for health problem. It is used for people who have a BMI 50 or more.

Section 4 Case reports on Simple Obesity Research by Acupuncture treatment
单纯性肥胖症针灸治疗研究进展验案

4.1 Modern Research
4.1.1 Body acupuncture

Obesity is caused by dysfunction of transportation and transformation of the body fluid, accumulation of dampness and phlegm turbidity, which are the result of disorders of Zang-Fu organs, stagnation of Qi and Blood, disharmony of the Thoroughfare and Conception vessels. Obesity achieved by needling meridian points to balance Yin and Yang, regulate Zang-Fu organs, promote flow of Qi and Blood of the meridians, and eliminates the pathogenic factors by dredging meridian and collateral. Needles can be twirled, electrically stimulated and left in place. The filiform needles with diameter of 0.25-0.30mm and length of 40-75mm were typically selected based on the case's obesity degree.

Meng et al. (Zhang, 2008) treated 180 cases of female simple obesity by using electro-acupuncture (EA) and 60 cases by manual acupuncture for controlling obesity. Ren 12, ST 25, Ren 4 and ST 36 were chosen as main points in both groups. In the EA treatment group, bilateral ST 25 was stimulated by electric device with disperse and dense wave and the strength bearable to patients. Needle were retained for 40 min. and the treatment was given 5 times a week followed by a 2 days interval in both group, and 20 sessions made up of a therapeutic course. The total effective rate of 97.8% and 88% was achieved in the EA treatment and control group respectively. Yin (Zhang, 2008) chose Ren 12, Ren 4, and SP 6 as main points, and added secondary points according to differentiation of symptoms and signs. After the arrival of Qi by lifting and thrusting for reinforcing and reducing, electric device was applied to the main points with continuous waves and 20/sec. in frequency and intensity tolerable to patients. The treatment was given once every other day, and 10 treatments made up a therapeutic course with an interval of 3 days between two courses of treatments was 87.5%.

As the function of the EA can be precisely characterized and the results are more or less copied, an attempt was made by Han Jisheng's research team to clarify whether EA of strictly identified parameters is effective to suppress the simple obesity induced by high energy diet in a rat model. In the diet induced obese rats, EA was applied at the posterior leg acupoints 3 times per week for 4 weeks with high energy diet and water provided. A significant reduction of the body weight accompanied by reduction in food intake was observed.

4.1.2 EA acupoint and its Frequency selection

2 Hz EA was more effective than 100 Hz EA (Tian et al., 2005). As its results, diet induced obese rats showed an increased level of plasma cholesterol and triglyceride. EA stimulation produced a reduction of

plasma level of total cholesterol and triglyceride. In this respect, 100 Hz EA was more effective than 2 Hz EA. If it is confirmed that 2 Hz EA is more effective in body weight loss and 100 Hz EA more effective in decreasing plasma lipid content, it may be worthwhile to try the 2/100 Hz alternative mode of stimulation to cover both sides of the disorder.

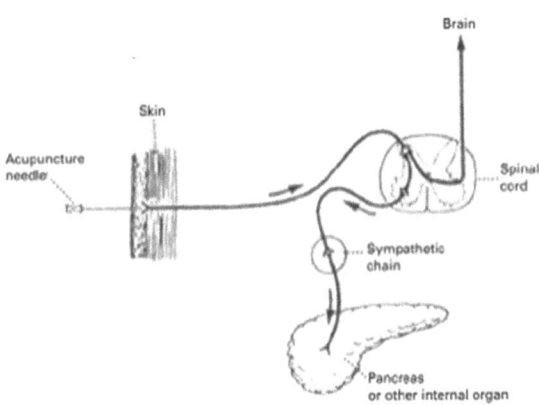

Figure 1 Simplified theoretical pathway of needle stimulation sending nerve impulses to brain and internal organ.[32]

Figure motivated from (10)

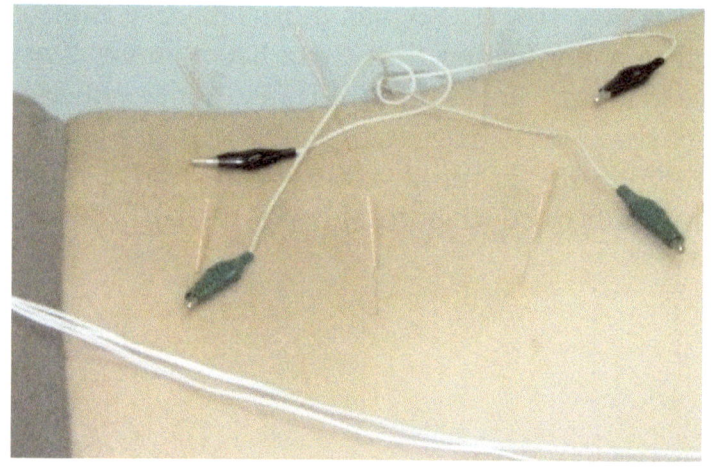

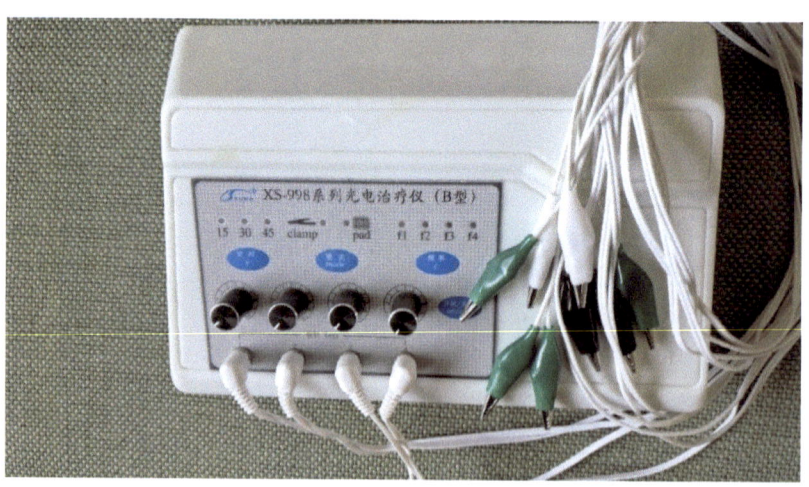

4.1.2 Auricular therapy

In TCM, the ears are an important pivot point for the meridians to communicate with each other. When the organs are in disharmony, it will be reflected on the ear. It produces dramatic body weight reductions in obese patients. It has physiologic and anorexigenic functions must be explained. Fetal somatotop and Nogier's inverted somatotopy have been analyzed. The similarity between the localization of the motor and somatosensory representations of the ear in the cerebral cortex in the fetus has also been noted in both Western and Chinese journals.

Apostolopoulos (26), Greece observed 800 cases; Auricular acupuncture (placement of press needles) was applied at the stomach point (according to Nogier) and sometimes at the point of psychological balance (Shenmen) for the control of anxiety and for help in weight loss in 800 patients over a two-year period. 683 women and 117 men aged between 15-76 years. There was significant weight loss in 64.8% and 35.5% at 6-12 months.

Press needles were inserted and left in for 10 to 15 days at the auricular acupuncture point and resided again after 4 to 5 days. At the same time, instructions were given for standard treatment of obesity including low calorie diet, aerobic exercise, behavior modification, psychological support etc. The patients were followed up for period of one year. The control of overeating and anxiety using auricular acupuncture at the stomach and Shenmen points has been beneficial. Auricular acupuncture on the stomach area and Shenmen which psychological balance point was employed for the control of overeating and anxiety and as an aid to weight loss in 800 individuals in the 1993-1994. Stomach point provokes a sensation of fullness after eating a small amount of food, and the therapeutic benefit lies in the inhibition of appetite, and not to be obese for a longer period. The stomach area is also called "root of the helix".

Shiraishi (40), Japan observed; 55 people which are male 26 and female 29, whom are healthy volunteers averaging 34.5 (17-57) years of age, with a BMI of 24.3 kg/m2 and 5 mildly obese patients; average age 31.6 years, BMI 26.5kg/m2. Small auricular needles (0.15 x2.0 mm) were inserted and replaced with new ones once every week. Body weight was measured four times a day which was immediately after waking in the morning, immediately after breakfast, and after dinner, and before going to bed. Experimental period were weeks 3 to 8 weeks.

There were 501 in group A (female 262, male 239) and 520 in group (female 261, male 259). Study was age, sex, and BMI respect to the experimental subjects. In group A measured their body weight for 18 weeks which were without any acupuncture related stimulation or interference with their ears. In group B measured their body weight four times a day, like group A. Group B received auricular needles intracutaneously into the bilateral cavum conchae once a week, in weeks 3 to 8 and 10 to 15. Group was measured body adipose, body weight, and waist-hip ratio. As a result, obese patient was most successful of losing weight. Daily body weight changes in the same patient, whose weight was significantly, reduced about 5 kg by 18 weeks with bilateral auricular acupuncture stimulation.

Selected acupoints for obesity are; Large Intestine, Small Intestine, Lung, Triple Burner, Endocrine, Subcortex, Hunger center, thirst center, constipation center, sympathetic, Stomach, Esophagus, Mouth, Adrenal gland and Spleen.

Hsieh CH (127) observed that 56 young adults who ranged in age from 18 to 20 years old for auricular acupressure on weight reduction and abdominal obesity for eight weeks with Japanese Magnetic Pearl for one group and another group got Semen Vaccariae on the ear acupoint. Both groups showed significant reductions to body weight and waist circumference after eight weeks of treatment. The group treated with Semen Vaccariae group showed a more effective weight loss for a short term. Auricular acupressure is a safe and cost-effective treatment for weight loss, and it is reasonable option for the treatment obesity for young people.

Selected acupoints for obesity are; Large Intestine, Small Intestine, Lung, Triple Burner, Endocrine, Subcortex, Hunger center, Thirst center, Constipation center, Sympathetic, Stomach, Esophagus, Mouth, Adrenal gland and Spleen.

Richards D (129) observed that 60 overweight people randomly divided into an active and a control group, used the AcuSlim device twice for four weeks. The active group was attached the device to the ear points Shenmen and stomach. The control group was attached the device to their thumb where was no acupuncture points. As the results, 95% of the active group reacted suppression of appetite, but control group was no reaction showed. Specific auricular acupuncture points are an effective method of appetite suppression for weight loss. Auricular acupuncture stimulates to the ear which vagal nerve and raises serotonin levels and they have been shown to increase tone in the smooth muscle of the stomach which is suppressing appetite.

Figure motivated from (44)

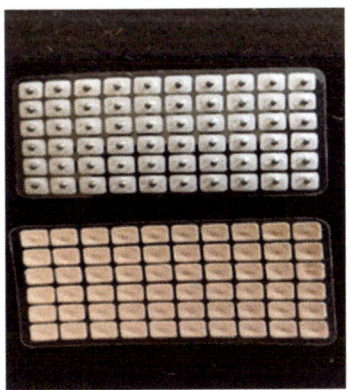

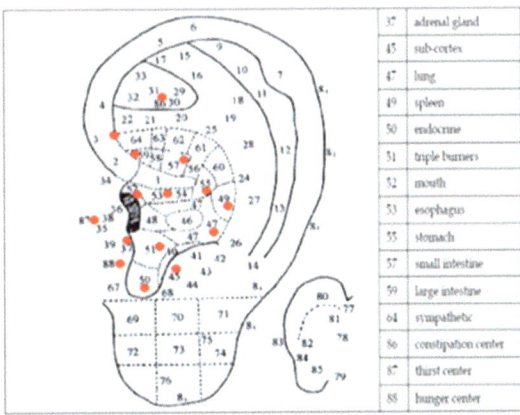

37	adrenal gland
45	sub-cortex
47	lung
49	spleen
50	endocrine
51	triple burners
52	mouth
53	esophagus
55	stomach
57	small intestine
59	large intestine
64	sympathetic
86	constipation center
87	thirst center
88	hunger center

Fig. 4. Selected aural acupoints in weight loss (ICMHL, Shen-Nong Info. e)

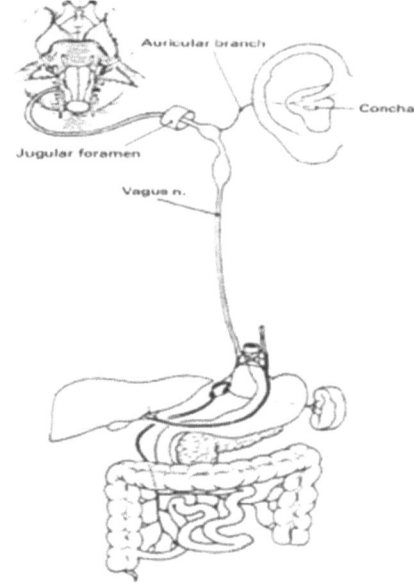

Figure 3   Scheme of distribution of the vagus nerve.

Figure motivated from (10)

4.1.3 Moxibution

Yang et al (Zhang, 2008) (44) used moxibution with warming needle to treat 32 cases of simple obesity of deficiency type by selecting Ren 6 (气海 Qihai), Ren 4 (关元 Guanyuan), ST 36 (足三里 Zusanli), ST 25 (天 枢), SP 9 (阴陵泉 Yinlingquan), and SP 6 (三阴交 Sanyinjiao) as the main points and secondary points according to differentiation of symptoms and signs. After the arrival of Qi, 1-2 lighted moxa sticks about 2cm in length were sequentially put on the handles of the needles of the 2-3 main points, and the other needles were retained as usual. The treatment was given 6 times weekly, and 30 sessions constituted a therapeutic course. A total effective rate of 90.6% was achieved after one course of treatment.

Shen Tao et al (161) observed 48 cases of obesity by cap-shaped warm acupuncture to treat obesity with hyperlipidemia using points of Du 20 (白会 Baihui), P 6 (內關 Naiguan), ST 36 (足三里 Zusanli), Liv 3 (太冲 Taichong), KI 7 (复瘤 Fuliu), Ren 4 (关元 Guanyuan), ST 25 (天枢 Tianshu) and Ren 12 (中脘 Zhongwan). After 4 courses treatment, 15 cases got marked effectiveness, 23 cases got effectiveness and 10 cases failed, and total effective rate was 79.2%.

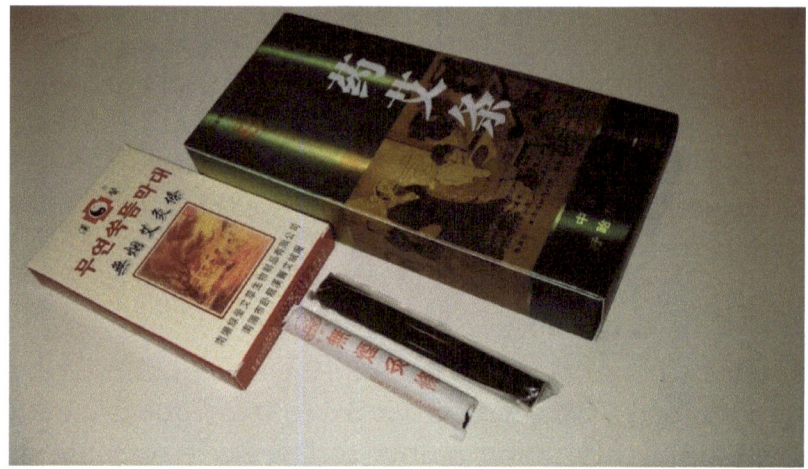

Moxa

4.1.4 Catgut Embedding therapy

Chen F et al (125) investigated the mechanism of acupoint catgut embedding in the treatment of simple obesity. 80 simple obesity patients were randomly and divided into acupoint catgut embedding group and acupuncture group. Acupoints selected on the basis of differentiation of symptoms and signs. ST 34 (梁丘 Liangqiu), Ren 12 (中脘 Zhongwan), ST 25 (天枢 Tianshu), Ren 9 (水分 Shuifen), ST 40 (丰隆 Fenglong) and Ashi point.

Catgut embedding was performed once a week and for 4 weeks therapeutic course. Acupuncture was given once a daily in the 1st 5 days, and once every other day. Before and after the treatment, body weight (BW) and body mass index (BMI) were found out. Fasting blood samples from ulnar vein for detecting insulin and glucose contents, and tumor necrosis factor concentration with enzyme linked immunosorbent test, and insulin resistance index. After the treatment, the two of 40 cases in acupuncture and acupoint catgut embedding groups, 12 and 13 were cured, and 13 and 15 had a marked improvement, 10 and 8 had an improvement, 5 and 4 failed. The effective rate was 87.5% and 90% respectively. There was not so much significant difference between the two groups.

Both acupoint catgut embedding and acupuncture have a definite therapeutic effect in the treatment of simple obesity, which is closely associated with the decline of serum insulin, glucose and tumor necrosis factor.

4.1.5 Other treatment
4.1.5 (1) Plum-Blossom Needle Therapy

Simple obesity of plum-blossom needle apply to the region where the subcutaneous fat is excessively deposited, such as the lumbar region and the abdominal region which are on both sides of the spinal column, the upper and lower abdominal regions, the anteromedial side of the leg, the inferior border of the mandible and ST 36 (足三里 Zusanli), SP 6 (三阴交 Sanyinjiao), Ren 12 (中脘 Zhongwan), P 6 (内关 Neiguan) and Du 14 (大椎 Dazhui) and the area of the positive masses. Modifications added to the upper back region, the lumbar region and the medial side of the leg, nape region, the sacral region, the liver region and the upper abdominal region. Moderate or heavy tappings should apply when the abdominal region receives tappings, the patient should stand erect and practice deep breathing.

Zhong Meiquan observed to a patient on simple obesity with 78kg on body weight and abdominal measurement was 111cm on plum-blossom needle. After one course of treatment by plum-blossom needle, the body weight reduced to 76kg, abdominal measurement to 105cm. After two courses of treatment, body weight reduced to 70kg. After 6 courses of treatment, body weight was further reduced to 62.5kg, abdominal measurement to 92cm.

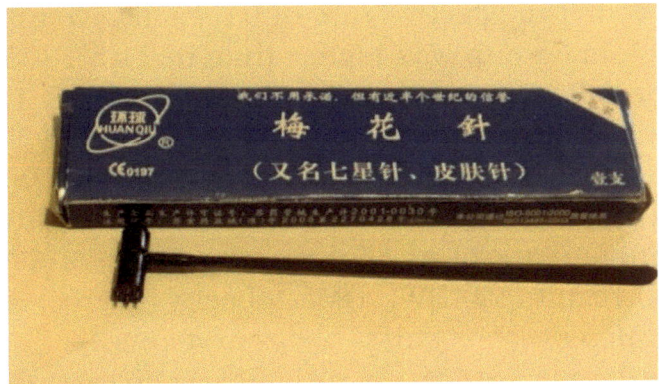

Plum-blossom needle

4.1.5 (2) Acupotomy

Chen M et al (46) at Nanjing Univ. Of TCM observed that 105 cases were randomly divided into an acupotomy group, an electroacupuncture group and an acupuncture group, 35 cases in each group. Ren 12 (中脘 Zhongwan), ST 25 (天枢 Tianshu), ST 37 (上

巨虚 Shangjuxu), SP 6 (三阴交 Sanyinjiao) etc., were selected in three groups and also with selection of acupoints according to symptoms. The acupotomy group was treated with acupotomy 40 mm in length and 0.6 mm in diameter, the electro-acupuncture group. The clinical therapeutic effects of three groups were compared, such as body weight (BW), body mass index (BMI), obesity degree, etc., and blood lipid and fasting blood sugar (FBS) were observed. The effective rate of 91.4% (32/35) in the acupotomy group was higher than of 71.5% (25/35) in the electroacupuncture group and of 42.9% (15/35) of body acupuncture group. It was better results of obesity signs and blood fat and fasting blood sugar (FBS) of the three groups after treatment for acupotomy group. Acupotomy group was also the better results of BW, BMI, obesity degree, chest circumference, waist circumference, thigh circumference, waist-hip ratio, total cholesterol after the treatment.

4.1.5 (3) Gua sha Therapy

Xiao Zhong ( ) investigated scraping for 30 times with point BL 23 (肾俞 Shenshu) on the back first, then scrape Ren 17 (膻中 Danzhong) on the chest, scrape the upper and lower parts of Ren 12 (中脘 Zhongwan), ST 25 (天枢 Tianshu), Ren 4 (关元 Guanyuan) on the abdomen, scrape SP 6 (三阴交 Sanyinjiao) in the inner side of lower limbs, finally scrape from ST 36 (足三里 Zusanli) to ST 40 (丰隆 Fenglong). It was effective result after treatment.

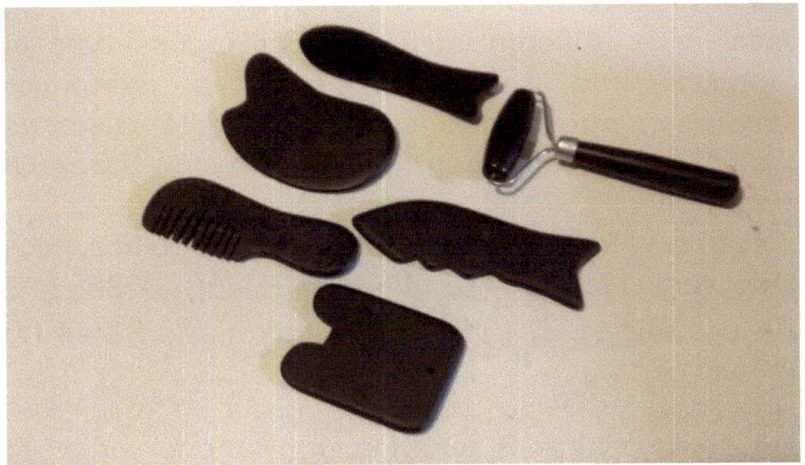

Gua sha made from Bianshi stone

4.1.6 Combination Therapy

4.1.6 (1) Body acupuncture and Ear treatment

Wei Qunli & Liu Zhicheng (140) investigated at Nanjing TCM university hospital the therapeutic effects of ear acupuncture, body acupuncture and the combined use of the two in the treatment of simple obesity, and 195 cases of obesity were divided into three groups, BA group (64 cases), EA group (55 cases), and BA + EA group (76 cases). Among the 140 cases (64+76) who received body acupuncture, 88 cases were differentiated as heat excess type of Stomach and Intestine, 34 cases dampness stagnation due to Spleen deficiency, 11 cases as Kidney Qi insufficiency, and 7 cases as Liver Qi stagnation.

For those whom Stomach and Intestine Heat excess type were selected with LI 4 (合谷 Hegu), ST 36 (足三里 Zusanli), ST 37 (上巨虚 Shangjuxu) and ST 44 (内庭 Neiting).

For those whom Stagnation of Dampness due to Spleen deficiency type were selected with ST 36 (Zusanli), ST 40 (丰隆 Fenglong), SP 6 (三阴交 Sanyinjiao), SP 9 (阴陵泉 Yinlingquan), Ren 12 (中脘 Zhongwan) and Ren 6 (气海 Qihai).

For patients who were insufficient Kidney Qi selected with BL 23 (肾俞 Shenshu), Ren 4 (关元 Guanyuan), SJ 6 (支沟 Zhigou) and KI 6 (照海 Zhaohai).

For those whom with Liver Qi stagnation were selected with BL 18 (肝俞 Ganshu), Liv 8 (曲泉 Ququan), GB 43 (侠溪 Xiaxi) and Liv 3 (太冲 Taichong). Needle was retained for 30 minutes, and the treatment was given once every other day. Twelve courses were for the treatment in all. For the 131 cases (55+76), who received ear acupuncture, 85 cases were differentiated as the Stomach and Intestine heat excess pattern, 31 cases were dampness stagnation due to Spleen deficiency, 9 cases as insufficient Kidney Qi, and 6 cases as Lever Qi stagnation.

For those whom were Stomach and Intestine heat excess, received ear points of Hunger, Endcrine, Lung and Shenmen. For those whom were dampness stagnation due to Spleen deficiency, received ear points of Spleen, Stomach, Endocrine and Lung. For those whom were Kidney Qi insufficient received ear points of Kidney, Sanjiao, Endocrine and Lung. For those whom were Liver Qi stagnation, received ear points Liver, Endocrine, Lung and Shenmen.

Therapeutic effects of body acupuncture and body acupuncture plus ear acupuncture were significantly better result than only ear acupuncture treatment. In final, most effectiveness was body acupuncture combined with ear acupuncture therapy.

4.1.6 (2) Body acupuncture and Moxibution

Shi et al (131) investigated the clinical effect of acupuncture-moxibution therapy on Simple Obesity due to Spleen deficient 68 cases of Simple Obesity of def. syndrome types, including internal Dampness due to Spleen def., Lung Q def., Spleen Qi def., Spleen Yang def., Kidney Yang def., were randomly set aside into 2 groups which are treatment group (36 cases) which was treated with warm needling moxibution,

and control group (32 cases) which was treated with electroacupuncture. Ren 12 (中脘 Zhongwan), Ren 9 (水分 Suifen), Ren 6 (气海 Qihai), Ren 3 (中级 Zhongji) and bilateral ST 25 (天枢 Tianshu), ST 28 (水道 Suidao), P 6 (内关 Neiguan), LI 4 (合谷 Hegu), SP10 (血海 Xuehai), ST 36 (足三里 Zusanli), ST 40 (丰隆 Fenglong), SP 6 (三阴交 Sanyinjiao) were chosen as main points in both groups.

Bilateral SP 15 (大橫 daheng), SP 14 (腹結 Fujie), SP 9 (阴陵泉 Yinlingquan), SP 4 (公孙 Gongsun), BL 20 (脾俞 Pishu), BL21 (胃俞 Weishu) and BL24 (气海俞 Qihaishu) were added as supplement acupoints of Dampness due to Spleen deficiency.

Bilateral LU 5 (尺泽 Chize), LU 7 (列缺 Lieque), SP 9 (阴陵泉 Yinlingquan), BL 13 (肺俞 Feishu), BL 20 (脾俞 Pishu), BL 43 (膏肓俞 Gaohuangshu) for Lung and Spleen of Qi deficiency.

Ren 4 (关元 GuanYuan), Du 4 (命门 Mingmen) and bilateral ST 29 (归来 Guilai), LI 10 (手三里 Shousanli), KI 3 (太溪 Taixi), KI 7 (复瘤 Fuliu), BL 20 (脾俞 Pishu), BL 23 (肾俞 Shenshu) were added for Spleen and Kidney of Yang deficiency.

Electro acupuncture apparatus were with continuous wave and at frequency of 2 Hz, by the intensity of stimulation within the patient's tolerance and favorite.

For warming needle moxibustion was done on 3-4 pairs acupoints for each pattern Ren 6 (气海 Qihai) and bilateral ST 28 (水道 Shuidao), SP 9 (阴陵泉 Yinlingquan), SP 6 (三阴交 Sanyinjiao) were selected for internal Dampness due to Spleen deficiency;

Ren 9 (水分 Shuifen) and bilateral LU 5 (尺泽 Chize), ST 36 (足三里 Zusanli), SP 6 (三阴交 Sanyinjiao) for Lung and Spleen Qi deficiency;

Ren 9 (水分 Shuifen), Ren 4 (关元 Guanyuan) and bilateral KI 3 (太溪 Taixi), ST 36 (足三里 Zusanli) for Spleen and Kidney Yang deficiency; Two cones of moxa roll with length of 1.5-2.0cm were inserted into the needle handle and light it. The needles were retained for 30 min. The treatment was done every other day and 15 times made up of a course. After one course of treatment, the therapeutic efficacy was analyzed and indicated that the weight loss value of treatment group was obviously higher than that electro acupuncture group.

It was shown that for treating Simple Obesity due to Spleen deficiency was by warming needle moxibustion method has more advantage than electro acupuncture method.

4.1.6 (3) Body acupuncture, Auricular treatment and Moving Cupping
Bu TW et al (128) observed that 80 cases divided into 3 groups.

The body acupuncture group was treated based on the syndrome of heat of stomach and intestine, syndrome of spleen deficiency and stagnation of dampness, and syndrome of spleen and kidney yang deficiency.

The body acupuncture and auricular group were treated by the syndrome treatment of body acupuncture combined with auricular point.

The third group was treated with by combination of body acupuncture, auricular and moving cupping on Back-shu points. The investigation was body weight (BW), BMI, body fat, blood lipid, and for clinically main symptoms before and after treatment. As the results, the effective rate was 69.6% in the body acupuncture group, 76.0% were in the body acupuncture and auricular group, and 90.6% were combined group which was the body acupuncture, auricular and moving cupping group with significant therapeutic effect.

4.1.6 (4) Body acupuncture with electronic device, moving cupping and catgut embedding

Shi Y et al (126) observed that 82 cases of simple obesity with stomach and intestine excess-heat were randomly dividedly into group A (40) and group B

(42). Body acupuncture with EA were applied with point Ren 12 (中脘 Zhongwan), Ren 10 (下脘 Xiawan) and Ren 6 (气海 Qihai) in the two groups. Catgut embedding and moving cupping at the channels of Ren, Du, SP, ST and BL were added in group A. Group B was only body acupuncture with electronic device. The therapeutic effect, main symptoms, BW, BMI, waist circumference (WC), hip circumference (HC), and waist-hip rate (WHR) were investigated. As the results of the total effective rate was 90.0% in Group A and 78.6% in the group B. Group A and B were significantly differencing in decreasing of BW, BMI, waist circumference, HC, and main symptoms between the two groups.

It is a better method for treatment by combined body acupuncture with electronic device, moving cupping and catgut embedding which can increase therapeutic effect on simple obesity of stomach and intestine excess heat.

4.1.6 (5) Body acupuncture, electro-acupuncture combined with photoelectric (laser) treatment Instrument

AI Bing-Wei et al (155) observed that 60 cases of simple obesity were randomly divided into two groups, 30 cases in each group. Treatment group were with photoelectric treatment instrument combined with acupuncture, and XS-998 electro-acupuncture device was placed at points of the abdomen together with the laser pads on Ren 8 (神阙 Shenque), Ren 9 (水分 Shuifen) or the fat area, or close to the Liver area of the patients. The control group was treated with acupuncture only, and their symptoms, signs and BMI before and after treatment were recorded into two groups. As the result, the symptom, signs and BMI were significantly improved in the treatment compared with the control group. Acupuncture combined with laser radiation on the abdomen is the therapeutic effect on simple obesity.

4.1.6 (6) Acupuncture combined with Cupping for Treatment

Li Yanshuang et al (110) observed that 52 cases of simple obesity were randomly divided into three groups. As the result, the total effective rate was 90.4% with acupuncture combined with cupping method.

Lili Wang et al (93) observed that 50 cases of simple obesity were randomly divided into two groups which were two men and 48 women, the age between 20 to 52 years old, and the duration was 6 months. Patients had especially on abdominal and thigh treatment. As the result, the total effective was 47 cases and the rate was 94%.

4.1.6 (7) Body acupuncture plus Tuina therapy

Shang Xiao-Li et al (158) observed that 98 cases of simple obesity of the patients were randomly divided into the two groups and 60 cases in group were treated with acupuncture therapy plus Tuina, and 38 cases in the control group were with single acupuncture treatment. As a result, the effective rate was 100% in the treatment group and 71.0% in the control group.

Li Li-qiu et al (159) observed that 60 cases of simple obesity of stomach-intestine excessive heat type were randomly divided into acupuncture plus Tuina group and single acupuncture group which 30 cases respectively. As a result, the total effective rate in acupuncture plus Tuina group was 90.0% and simple acupuncture group was 73.3%.

4.1.6 (8) Body acupuncture plus massage

Xia Bo et al (160) reported that Dr. Guan Zun-hui observed 80 cases of simple obesity patients were randomized into two groups which 40 cases were treated by acupuncture and massaging abdomen with salt, and control group were 40 cases treated. As a result, the clinical cure rate and marked effective rate in treatment group were significantly higher in control group (P<0.01).

4.2 Progress in Mechanism Research
4.2.1 The role of the Central Nervous System

(1) Cerebral Cortex, Amygdala research
Liu Zhicheng et al (133) observed that body weight, body fat, and monoamine content of amygdala in obesity model of male SD rats obtained by high fat diet were observed before and after acupuncture. As a result, content of tyrosine (Tyr), dopamine (DA) and noradrenaline (NA) were lower in control group than those of normal, but the contents of serotonin (5 HT) and 5 HT/5 hydroxyindo leacetic acid (5 HIAA) were higher than those of normal. After the treatment by acupuncture, the weight loss was succeeding while the level of tyrosine (Tyr) and dopamine (DA) increased, and the level of serotonin (5 HT) and 5 HT/5 hydroxyindoleacetic acid (HIAA) decreased in

amygdale of obese rats. It has shown that a good regulative effect of acupuncture on amygdale of obese rat is an important link in the anti-obesity. Cholecyctokinin-octapeptide (CCK-8) is one of the brain-gut peptides widely distributed in neurons of the Central Nervous system, especially in cerebral cortex and hippocampus, and this peptide is a neurotransmitter.

Liu Zhichen et al (146) observed that the effects of acupuncture on the neurorchemical information mass in cerebral cortex of obese rats. The change of the body mass, index, body fat, and the contents of 5 hydroxytryptamine (5-HT), cholecystokinin (CCK) and vasoactive intestinal polypeptide (VIP) in the cerebral cortex of the obese rats were observed in the three groups before and after acupuncture. The results show that the obese rats were the contents of hydroxytryptamine (5-HT), colecystokinin (CCK) and VIP in the cerebral cortex were lower than normal rats. After the treatment by acupuncture, the body mass index was achieved and the contents of hydroxytryptamine (5-HT), cholecystokinin (CCK) and vasoactive intestinal polypeptide (VIP) were obviously increased in the cerebral cortex of the obese rats. He observed the good regulation of acupuncture on the contents of hydroxytryptamine (5-HT), cholecystokinin (CCK) and vasoactive intestinal polypeptide (VIP) in cerebral cortex of organism is possibly an important central mechanism in the anti-obesity of acupuncture.

(2) Hypothalamic Nuclei research

Liu Zhicheng et al (136) observed that effect of acupuncture on obese rats, and the obese parameters and the change of monoamines transmitters and activity of adenosine triphosphatase (ATP) in lateral hypothalamic area (LHA) of obese rats. As the results, the level of noradrenaline (NA) in lateral hypothalamic area (LHA) of obese rats were higher than in the normal group, but the level of serotonin (5-HT) and the activity of ATPase in LHA of obese rats were lower than the normal rats. After acupuncture treatment, the obese rats obtained reduced weight, meanwhile the level of noradrenaline (NA) in lateral hypothalamic area (LHA) was reduced and the serotonin (5-HT), and activity of ATPase was increased ($P<0.05$, $P<0.01$).

Liu Zhicheng et al (139) also observed that Spontaneous discharges of nerve cells in ventromedial neucleus of hypothalamus (VNH) and levels of monoamine neurotransmitters in obese rats by effective acupuncture treatment. The result was level of tyrosine (Tyr) and dopamine (DA) was decreased, and the levels of 5-hydroxytryptamine (5–HT) and 5–hydroxyindole acetic acid (5– HIAA) increased in ventromedial neucleus of hypothalamus (VNH). The spontaneous discharges of nerve cells in VNH lowered, spontaneous discharges of nerve cells in the VNH increased, and the levels of Tyr, DA, tryptamine, and 5–HT/5–HIAA increased, and 5–HT level decreased in VNH tissue. It is good regulative action of acupuncture on VNH is possibly one of the important factors for acupuncture in reducing body weight.

Zhao Mei et al (135) studied and showed that the effect of acupuncture on the feeding center of hypothalamus in fat rats. It was used for recording electric activities in unit time in the hunger center of lateral area of hypothalamus (LHA) and the satiety center of ventromedial nucleus of hypothalamus (VMH). As results, acupuncture can significantly reduce to excite of LHA, and increase frequency of electric activity in ventromedial nucleus of hypothalamus (VMH) and inhibit hyperorexia and reduce caloric intake for reducing fatty. So that, the regulative action of acupuncture on the central nuclei is reducing fatty that the main mechanisms of acupuncture.

Ma Cheng & Liu Zhicheng et al (138) observed that by changing of gastric function induced by the excitation of the lateral hypothalamus (LHA, the feeding center) by treatment of acupuncture, and research on the mechanism of the acupuncture to inhibit the excessive appetite and reduce hunger in obese people. EA at ST 36 (足三里 Zusanli) or ST 44 (内廷 Neiting) inhibit the hyperactive of the stomach induced by stimulation of LHA. As a result, electro acupuncture on ST 36 (足三里 Zusanli) obviously inhibits gastric hyperfunction by the excitation of the LHA. Thus, electro acupuncture effects through gastric β receptor, hence, inhibits the appetite, alleviates hunger, and reduces the body weight.

4.2.2 The role of Peripheral Nervous System
Liu Zhicheng et al (145) observed the obese rats of the levels of central and peripheral and the spontaneous discharges frequency of nerve cell in the Arcuate nucleus (ARC) in hypothalamus of obese

rats were observed before and after acupuncture. As the results, the effective weight loss was achieved with acupuncture treatment while levels of serum leptin and insulin (INS) obviously decreased, and the level of hypothalamic leptin and insulin (INS), and the spontaneous discharges frequency of nerve cell in ARC of obese rats were markedly increased. The good regulation function of acupuncture on the leptin and insulin (INS) levels of central and peripheral, and the nerve function of ARC were one of the anti-obesity mechanisms of acupuncture.

4.2.3 The role of Endocrine System

Thyroid disease is most often for causing obesity, especially adolescents. Richard Atkinson (107) observed in his patients who onset of weight gain at the same time with symptoms of hyperthyroidism, and with elevated thyroid hormone levels and depressed thyroid stimulating hormone (TSH) levels. Thyroid disease is commonly found in obese patients. glucocorticoid treatment is also common form of endocrine obesity. Weight gain with both glucocorticoid treatments will be large range of about 25-50kg weight loss. Weight gain of these levels in nature appears Cushing disease, which is pituitary tumor or Cushing syndrome due to adrenal adenoma.

Insulinoma is another rare case of causing from endocrine obesity. Endocrine diseases are treatable conditions, so that it significantly improves weight loss for patients.

Liu Zhicheng (147) observed in clinical on treatment of gastrointestinal excess heat type of 718 patients with simple obesity. It has achieved the effect of weight loss by acupuncture. It has shown that acupuncture had a good regulatory effect on the function of nerve and endocrine, digestion and energy metabolism.

4.2.4 The role of the level of Gene expression

Liu Zhicheng et al (143) observed that effect of acupuncture can increase the level of hypothalamic leptin in obese rats. The results show that after acupuncture treatment the level of serum leptin decreased, and the level of hypothalamic leptin increased in obese rats. The good regulation function of acupuncture on the levels of central and peripheral and the nerve function of ARC were one of the anti-obesity mechanisms of acupuncture.

Yang Chun-Zhuang et al (148) observed that the effect of electro acupuncture (EA) on serum leptin contents and the expression of leptin receptor in the hypothalamus in simple obesity rats. As the results, electro acupuncture (EA) can lower serum leptin level and regulate the expression of Leptin receptor in the hypothalamus in obesity rats.

Liu Zhicheng et al (151) investigated that the effects of acupuncture on the expression of uncoupling protein 1 (UCP1) gene of brown adipose tissue (BAT) in obese rats. Observations of obese rats were before and after acupuncture. As the results, the effect of weight loss was achieved by acupuncture, and the expression of UCP1 gene of brown adipose tissue (BAT) increased obviously in obese rats. The cause of obesity is the abnormal reduction for expression of UCP1 in obese organism which is an important cellular and molecular mechanism in anti-obesity effect by acupuncture.

4.2.5 The impact on Metabolism
4.2.5 (1) Glucose Metabolism
Liu. Zhicheng et al (143) observed that the effect of acupuncture on the contents and blood-brain transport of leptin and insulin in obese organism. As

the results, acupuncture can regulate on levels of hypothalamic and serum Leptin and Insulin and this is an important link in improving the resistance of leptin and insulin and regulate abnormal metabolism in obese organism.

Mehmet T Cabioglu et al (132) investigated that the effects of electro acupuncture (EA) on levels of serum insulin, c-peptide and glucose in obese women. The result that electro acupuncture (EA) is an effective method in treating obesity, and it helps also serum glucose levels to decrease through the increase of serum insulin and c-peptide levels.

4.2.5 (2) The function of Lipid Metabolism
Gao Jian-zhi et al (108) observed that the effect of acupuncture on lipid metabolism in simple obese rat and investigated the mechanism of acupuncture in weight reduction and providing evidence. As a result, obese rats with acupuncture decreased obviously the body weight and index. By treatment of acupuncture, the obese rat obtained for decreasing of the level of triglyceride (TG), total cholesterol (TC) and very low-density lipoprotein (VLDL)-ch, and the level of HDL-ch. Acupuncture works to decrease the

decomposition of lipid through the loss of energy intaking and more lipid produce energy to achieve weight loss.

Liu Zhicheng et al (149) observed that the effects of lipid reducing, and also some lipid disorders among obese patients. As a result, acupuncture treatment reduced of lipid, body fat, weight index, triglyceride (TG), free fat acid (FFA), very low-density lipoprotein (VLDL) and total cholesterol (TC) decreased significantly and basal metabolic rate (BMR) increased obviously after the treatment.

Cheng Ling et al (152) investigated that the effects and regulative function of acupuncture in obese patients. The results that acupuncture improved the parameters in body fat and regulate abnormal lipid metabolism in obese patients.

Wang SJ et al (163) observed the effect of high frequency electroacupuncture on lipid metabolism in 51 obesity rats. As a result, serum triglyceride (TG), total cholesterol (TC), low density lipid-cholesterol (LDL-C), fat weight, adipose cell area, serum leptin and insulin levels decreased significantly by electroacupuncture. High frequency EA can effectively improve abnormal lipid metabolism and reduce fat accumulation in obesity rats.

4.2.6 The role of the Digestive function
Liu Zcheng et al (147) investigated that the effects of acupuncture with Stomach-Intestine excess heat in obese patients. As a result, the weight loss effects were achieved by acupuncture. Acupuncture had a good effect on function of digestion. His clinical study also indicated that the salivary diastase, serum pepsinogen, serum amylase and urine D-xylose levels of those with simple obesity of the pattern of excessive heat in gastrointestine which indexes were significantly reduced by acupuncture treatment so that acupuncture inhibits excessive gastrointestinal digestion.

Section 5 Clinical Research
临床研究

5.1 Case Selection (Clinical data)
5.1.1 Western medicine diagnostic criteria
WHO has developed action plans for the global strategy on diet, physical activity and health in connection with obesity.

According to the World Health Organization (WHO), the obesity is classified into class 3.

Table 1 WHO obesity classification using BMI values

BMI	Classification	BSMI (for Asian)	Risk of comorbidities
<18.5	Underweight	<18.5	Low (but risk of other clinical problems increased)
18.5 – 24.9	Normal weight	18.5 – 22.9	Average
25.0 – 29.9	Pre-obese (overweight)	23.0 – 24.9	Increased
30.0 – 34.9	Obese class 1	25.0 – 29.9	Moderate
35.0 – 39.9	Obese class 2	≥30.0	Severe
≥ 40.0	Obese class 3		Very severe

Table 2 Waist circumference (cm)

Comorbidity risk	Women	Men
Above action level 1	≥80	≥94
Above action level 2	≥88	≥102

Clinically, the diagnosis of obesity is that it takes place of:

- History of illness, physical examination and laboratory test excluding secondary obesity.
- BMI greater than or equal to 25 is overweight and 30 is obesity considered by WHO.
- Body weight Index (BMI): is a simple index of weight-for-height and used to classify overweight and obesity in adults.
- Standard weight (kg) = (height (cm) – 100) x 0.9
- Body fat (F %): Total body fat weight/total body weight (visceral or subcutaneous deposition of fat).

5.1.2 TCM diagnostic criteria

According to WHO, it was further discussion of obesity which diagnosis of simple obesity, and its evaluation standard are as follows:

- Spleen Dampness type: obesity, edema, fatigue, body weight difficulties, oliguria, anorexia, thin pulse, thin greasy tongue, red color.
- Gastro-Intestinal heat pattern: obesity, distention, dizziness, lethargy, thirst, enjoy drinking, slippery pulse, yellow greasy tongue.
- Liver Qi stagnation pattern: obesity, pain in chest, fullness of epigastric, irregular

menstruation, amenorrhea, insomnia, string pulse, white greasy tongue, dark red tongue.

- Spleen deficiency pattern: obesity, fatigue, weakness, back pain, impotence, feels cold, thin and string pulse, greasy tongue, and red tongue.
- Yin deficiency pattern: obesity, dizziness, headache, back & knee pain, hot in body, low fever, rapid and thin pulse, thin and red tongue.

5.2 Method of treatment

It was divided two groups out of 60 cases in details as follows:

1. Electro-acupuncture combined with laser group was 30 cases.
2. Electro-acupuncture group was also 30 cases.

5.2.1 Electro-acupuncture combined with laser group Treatment

Main Acupuncture Points:

ST 25 (天枢 Tianshu), Ren 9 (水分 Shuifen), Ren 12 (中脘 Zhongwan), Ren 6 (气海 Qihai), Ren 4 (关元 Guanyuan), ST 28 (水道 Suidao), SP 14 (腹結 Fujie),

SP 15 (大橫 Daheng), GB 26 (带脉 Daimai), LI 4 (合谷 Hegu), LI 11 (曲池 Quchi), SJ 6 (支沟 Zhigou), SP10 (血海 Xuehai), SP 11 (箕们 Jimen), ST 32 (伏兔 Futu), SP 6 (三阴交 Sanyinjiao), ST 36 (足三里 Zusanli), ST 44 (内廷 Neiting), SP 15 (大橫 Daheng),

5.2.2 Electro-acupuncture group treatment

Main and dialectical points, location of the points and operation methods are the same as electro-acupuncture combined with laser group.

Method of Operation:

It was applied with sterilized cotton on point of the skin of the patient's body. Needles were used sterilized one-time use, and the size of needle was 0.30 x 40mm Hua Tuo Brand. It was punctured perpendicularly into the point quickly. It was used reinforcing and reducing method in order to the patient's symptom and acceptance. After that it was applied with electro device, XS-998 which was produced by Nanjing Komatsu Medical Research Institute, on the both side of point of ST 25 (天枢 Tianshu), ST 28 (水道 Shuidao), Ren 9 (水分 Shuifen), Ren 12 (中脘 Zhongwan), SP 14 (腹結 Fujie). Intensity of strength of the device was depended on patient's tolerance. Needle and electro-acupuncture device were remained for 30 minutes for every day, and 10 times per course of treatment, intermittent one day to the next course of treatment. At the same time of performing with electro-acupuncture, was applied laser treatment with low power, output power 5mw, and wave 650nn on the area of Liver.

Statistical Methods

SPSS17.0 statistical method was used for data statistics including the measurement of persons and the standard deviation: before and after treatment compared with test, and data was used x^2 test.

Results

- ### Status of Patients

Table 1 General situation of patients in each group

Group	Number of cases	Male	Female	BMI	Age	VFA
Electro-acupuncture plus laser group	30	6	24	31.23±3.85	28.03±6.40	94.00±16.32
Electro-acupuncture group	30	5	25	30.53±2.96	33.17±10.80	90.67±18.56

Comparison of the two groups in gender, BMI, age, VFA and significant difference in statistic was (P>0.05).

- **Change of the Index before and after treatment**

Table 2. Electro-acupuncture plus laser indicator changes of before and after treatment

Index	Before treatment	After treatment
Body weight	87.90±17.13	76.70±14.39
Waist circumference	99.87±10.54	91.17±9.15
Hip circumference	110.10±8.21	102.30±7.15
Thigh circumference	62.63±4.82	58.93±4.54
BMI (Body mass index)	31.00±4.00	27.40±3.42
FAT (Body fat percentage)	36.64±3.87	32.54±3.75
VFA (Visceral fat)	94.00±16.32	75.67±11.94

Comparison by T test: Before and after of electro-acupuncture plus laser treatment group was measured body weight, waist, hip, thigh circumstance, BMI, FAT and VFA. Significant difference in statistic was (P<0.01).

Table 3 Electro-acupuncture (EA) indicator changes before and after treatment

Index	Before treatment	After treatment
Body weight	82.17±9.60	74.00±8.57
Waist circumference	98.87±8.14	92.33±7.24
Hip circumference	109.60±5.24	102.03±4.85
Thigh circumference	64.60±3.71	60.77±3.32
BMI (Body mass index)	30.20±2.72	27.14±2.51
FAT (Body fat percentage)	36.86±3.50	33.43±3.24
VFA (visceral fat)	90.67±18.56	78.67±15.70

Comparison by T test: Before and after of electro-acupuncture alone group was measured body weight, waist, hip, thigh circumstance, BMI, FAT and VFA. Significant difference in statistic was (P<0.01).

Table 4 Changes index after treatment

Index	Electro acupuncture plus laser group	EA group	Probability (P) value
Body weight	11.20±6.28	8.17±2.53	0.017
Waist circumference	8.70±2.97	6.53±2.11	0.002
Hip circumference	7.80±235	7.57±1.57	0.653
Thigh circumference	3.70±1.99	3.83±1.21	0.754
BMI (Body mass index)	3.60±1.28	3.06±0.93	0.067
FAT (Body fat percentage	4.10±1.15	3.43±1.08	0.024
VFA (Visceral fat)	18.33±9.50	12.00±4.84	0.002

Comparison by T test: Body weight, FAT was significantly decreased and probability (P<0.05). VFA was shown highly significant difference (P<0.01). Two groups of BMI, hip and thigh circumference was decreased, but it was not much difference in statistical number. As a result, it was shown that electro-acupuncture combined with laser in reducing body fat rate (FAT), waist circumference and visceral fat (VFA) was more effective than EA group alone in simple obesity.

Comparison of efficacy of treatment in two groups before and after weight loss

Table 1   Comparison of efficacy in two groups of weight loss

Group	Recovery	Markedly effective	Effective	Failed	Total effective rate (%)
Electro-acupuncture combined with laser group	1	12	14	3	90.00
EA group	1	5	21	3	90.00

As a result, the above-mentioned table 1 was shown that method of electro-acupuncture combined with laser group were apparently more effective than electro-acupuncture alone group regarding the point of view of the therapeutic effectiveness, but comparison of total effectiveness was P>0.05 and this was not the difference statistically significant.

5.2.3 Point selection

In clinically, when patients are differentiated in obesity, it is shown that they have symptom of excess heat of stomach and intestine, dampness and phlegm of spleen dysfunction, metabolism of spleen and kidney, Qi stagnation and so on. Therefore, treatment should be stomach, spleen, and especially spleen dysfunction is the key to the pathogenesis.

It is therefore four channels select for weight loss such as Stomach, Spleen, Bladder and Ren channel. It is used essential points and added from chosen points along according to the symptom. When there is certain place of fatness, then it is used Ashi points.

Mainly by taking these points to adjust the gastrointestinal absorption and metabolism function, adjust the endocrine, to achieve lipid lower and lose weight.

5.2.4 Basic points

As many ancient well-known physicians in China had been discovered and informed in written in the classical texts as obesity should concern spleen, Qi, phlegm and dampness. Spleen dysfunction is the key to the pathogenesis of this disease such as the spleen lost the circulation in the body, stagnation, and then produces phlegm in the body, and then it will build up in visceral fat and on the skin to be obesity. Therefore, the treatment should be done to spleen and stomach by focusing on specific points which related to this area in order to reduce the body weight.

It can be always used essential points group such as ST 25 (天枢 Tianshu), Ren 9 (水分 Shuifen), Ren 12 (中脘 Zhongwan), Ren 6 (气海 Qihai), Ren 4 (关元 Guanyuan), ST 28 (水道 Shuidao), SP 14 (腹结 Fujie), SP 15 (大横 Daheng), GB 26 (带脉 Daimai), LI 4 (合谷 Hegu), LI 11 (曲池 Quchi), SJ 6 (支沟 Zhigou), SP10 (血海 Xuehai), SP 11 (箕门 Jimen), ST 32 (伏兔 Futu), SP 6 (三阴交 Sanyinjiao), ST 36 (足三里 Zusanli), ST 44 (内廷 Neiting) and SP 15 (大横 Daheng) together with dialectical points if necessary.

Using the above all combined these points, it is helping for Spleen dampness, Phlegm, intestinal organs, digestive, to excrete humidity from the body in order to be smooth Qi circulation and adjusting in the whole body.

5.2.5 Dialectical points

Simple Obesity has often clinically categorized from relating the visceral reasons.

In obesity, it is said that important to pay attention for the dysfunction of Stomach and Intestine, Spleen, Kidney and Liver Qi because they seem to be a kind of mechanism of disease. Spleen is one of an important Zang organ, and if it happened to become dysfunction, water would be stagnated, and it finally causes to get dampness and phlegm in the body. Liver Qi stagnation which relates with the emotional factors and it finally ends to the Kidney dysfunction in water metabolism.

In obesity treatment, as there is relation to the dysfunction, the pathological mechanism, deficiency and stagnation, thus it will be differentiated as follows;

(1) Stomach and Intestine Excess heat type

Manifestation; heavy, excessive appetite, diet, sweet, fatty, greasy, salty, fried, lot of cold water. Dislike heat, dry stool, constipation, tongue red, yellow coating, pulse wiry, slippery, rapid. More than 80% of patients in obese have these symptoms.

(1) Dampness due to Spleen deficiency

Manifestation; accumulating phlegm, Spleen function is no good. Poor appetite, lassitude, heaviness due to dampness, abdominal distension, loose stool, scanty urine, edema in limbs in some cases, tongue body pale, swollen, tender, tongue coating is thin, greasy, various colour, pulse is deep, thready, sleeping pulse.

(2) Liver Qi stagnation

Manifestation; heavy body, distension, fullness of hypochondria region, emotional problem, depression, irritability, insomnia, irregular menstruation (including irregular cycle, alternative cycle, longer, shorter, no menstruation, amenorrhea), colour is dark, black colour, tongue coating is white, thin coating and greasy. Pulse is thready and wildly.

(3) Spleen and Kidney Yang deficiency

Manifestation; heavy body, Kidney deficiency, lumber soreness, Yin and Yang Qi deficiency, Spleen Yang deficiency, no energy, weakness, lassitude, cold, aversion to cold limbs, facial puffiness, loose stool, abdominal distension, impotent, cold uterus. Tongue coating pale, thin, greasy, large & swollen, pulse deep, thready, weak

(4) Liver and Kidney Yin deficiency

Manifestation; Heavy body, dizziness, blurred vision, distending headache, lumber pain (kidney deficiency), hot sensation, fever in afternoon (low), tongue flat red (tip red), little coating because heat, dry without moisture, pulse thready, thin rapid (heat inside), slightly wiry.

(1) Eliminate Heat and promote Stomach and Intestine:

On the first, eliminate and clear heat, and promote digestion.

Hand and Foot of Yangming meridian, that is, Stomach and Intestine points are most suitable for obese person who has symptoms, such as constipation, sweating, hunger and yellow urine and tongue. Points are LI-11(曲池 Quchi), LI-4 (合谷 Hegu), ST 21 (梁门 Liangmen), ST 44 (内廷 Neiting).

The three points such as LI 4 (合谷 Hegu) which is Yuan source point of Large Intestine, LI 11 (曲池 Quchi) and ST 36(足三里 Zusanli) are the main points and ST 44 (内廷 Neiting) as supplement. These three points can strongly reduce excess heat and clear fire of heat. However, ST 36 (足三里 Zusanli) which He-Sea point of Stomach and ST 44 (内廷 Neiting) which is water point of Stomach, thus these three points are as main point for the patient of inhibiting appetite and to improve their resistance of Insulin. Ma Cheng and Liu Zhicheng (138) observed and showed the evidence of electro-acupuncture at ST 36 (足三里 Zusanli) or ST 44 (内廷 Neiting) could inhibit the hyperactivity from the stomach induced by stimulation of hypothalamus area (LHA). By using method of electro-acupuncture on ST 36 (足三里 Zusanli) has an anticholinergic effect through the gastric β receptor, therefore inhibits appetite, and then patients gradually do not feel hungry, thus body weight in obesity will be reduced. Cheng et al (152) observed and showed evidence of ST 36 (足三里 Zusanli) combination with the other points, improved the situation of insulin resistance in patients with simple obesity. ST 21 (梁们 Liangmen) is an important point of digestion.

It is always to use the points such as ST 36 (足三里 Zusanli) and ST 37 (上巨虚 Shangjuxu) and especially when the patient has main symptom of constipation due to excess heat, it can be used ST 36 (足三里 Zusanli), ST 37 (上巨虚 Shangjuxu) which is lower He-Sea point of Large Intestine and also can add ST 39 (下巨虚 Xiajuxu) which is lower He-Sea point of Small Intestine for cool down the heat, and these three points are effective for this situation. It can also inhibit appetite and promote the movement of digestion in stomach and intestine. If the patient feels thirsty very much, ST 34 (梁丘 Liangqiu) which is Xi-cleft of stomach channel.

(2) Regulate function of Stomach and Spleen:

Stomach and spleen are the acquired essence. Spleen is one of the Zang organs for manufacture of Qi and Blood. Dysfunction of Stomach and Spleen lead in fail to transform and transport of foods and drinks, and it finally causes to descend Stomach Qi and ascend Spleen Qi in failure. It leads also deficiency of Qi and Blood. In these cases, ST 36 (足三里 Zusanli), SP 6 (三阴交 Sanyinjiao) and ST 44 (内

廷 Neiting) is related for Stomach and Spleen meridian, and besides regulate Qi, Blood, and Yin, Yang with reinforcing or reducing of methods.

ST 37 (上巨虚 Shangjuxu), ST 39 (下巨虚 Xiajuxu) and BL 11 (大杼 Dazhu) can be added for regulate of Qi and Blood. SP 10 (血海 Xuehai) and BL 17 (膈俞 Geshu) are for regulating Blood. ST 36 (足三里 Zusanli), Ren 6 (气海 Qihai) and Ren 12 (中脘 Zhongwan) can be added for strengthen of Qi in case of deficiency of Qi (Wei Qi) which originates from the stomach and derived from Qi of food essence, and Wei Qi circulates outside of vessels. ST 25 (天枢 Tianshu) can also be added. SP 6 (三阴交 Sanyinjiao) can be treated for diabetes II patients in obesity as SP 6 (三阴交 Sanyinjiao) regulates insulin excretion properly and elevates the level of insulin in blood plasma. ST 29 (归来 Guilai) can be added for regulate menstruation if necessary. ST 40 (丰隆 Fenglong) which is Luo-connection point, can use for dampness and phlegm symptom of patient.

(3) Nourish Kidney Qi and making smooth water metabolism:

When the deficiency of Kidney Q, it comes normally from weakness of Stomach and Spleen, and it finally become dysfunction of water metabolism. In such case, ST 36 (足三里 Zusanli) and SP 9 (阴陵泉 Yinlingquan) are He-sea points of water of Stomach and Spleen meridian. SP 9 (阴陵泉 Yinlingquan) is especially good point for edema in case of symptoms of patient. For tonify the Kidney Qi, SJ 6 (支沟 Zhigou) and KI 6 (照海 Zhaohai) are selected as addition. KI 3 (太溪 Taixi) which can work for dry throat and heat in the mouth with saliva if the patient feels for thirst. Both of KI 3 (太溪 Taixi) and KI 6 (照海 Zhaohai) are good point for Yin deficiency for patient. Ren 4 (关元 Guanyuan), BL 23 (肾俞 Shenshu) and BL 20 (脾俞 Pishu) can be added with reinforcing method for the patient feels lassitude due to Kidney Qi deficiency. SP 9 (阴陵泉 Yinlingquan) has function of opening and moving the water passages, and it is effective of enuresis for the patient in relation with Kidney deficiency.

(3)-1 Yang deficiency of Spleen and Kidney

It can be used point BL 20(脾俞 Pishu), BL 23 (肾俞 Shenshu), Ren 4 (气海 Qihai), SP 9(阴陵泉 Yinlingquan).

(3)-2 Yin deficiency of Spleen and Kidney

It can be used point BL 18(肝俞 Ganshu), BL 23(肾俞 Shenshu), KI 3(太溪 Taixi) and KI 6 (照海 Zhaohai).

(4) Calming Liver and regulate Qi:

Liver and Heart channel were selected as main points. Liv 3 (太冲 Taichong), Liv 2 (行间 Xingjian), GB 34 (阳陵泉 Yanglingquan) and BL 18 (肝俞 Ganshu) was chosen for this case to reduce fire and heat. GB 34 (阳陵泉 Yanglingquan) can soothe Liver and Gall Bladder. If the patent has symptom of borborygmus or regurgitation, then BL 21 (胃俞 Weishu) which is stomach of Back-shu point is a good point for patient in obese. If patient has symptom of insomnia, then HT 7 (神门 Shenmen) to be add, and SP 6 (三阴交 Sanyingjiao) may be used for in any time in obese patient.

(4)-1 Severe and heavy Syndrome:

If the patient shows that the syndrome is severe condition such as constipation, insomnia, abdominal distention and shortness of breath or palpitation, it can be used points as;

Constipation can be used points of SJ 6 (支沟 Zhigou) to clear heat and move the stool, ST 39 (下巨虚 Xiajuxu) of lower He-Sea point, KI 6 (照海 Zhaohai) to regulate lower jiao and BL 57 (承山 Chengshan) to control constipation and bowel movement.

Insomnia can be used points of KI 6 (照海 Zhaohai) and BL 62 (申脉 Shenmai) for Yin and Yang balance. The Spiritual Pivot states that Bladder channel enter the brain and divided into Yin and Yang, thus Yin and Yang meets in this point.

Abdominal detention can be used points of BL 27 (小肠俞 Xiaochangshu) of Back-Shu point of Small Intestine which regulates the Intestines and Bladder and ST 39 (下巨虚 Xiajuxu) of lower He-Sea point of Small Intestine to moves Small Intestine Qi and transforms stagnation.

Shortness of breath or palpitation symptom can be used the points of HT 7 (神门 Shenmen) of Yuan-Source for calming sprit and regulate the heart and P 6 (内关 Neiguan) of Luo-connecting point for harmonizing the chest with agitation of palpitation.

(4)-2 Efficacy of Laser

Laser is as the stimulation of traditional Chinese acupuncture points with low-intensity laser irradiation. This therapeutic use of laser acupuncture is rapidly gained in popularity. It is controlled by parameters such as wavelength and by skin properties such as pigmentation and thickness. The depth of laser energy transmission is an important to determine efficacy. Laser acupuncture reduce calorie diet, body weight, BMI and visceral for obesity. Laser acupuncture is uninfected, painless stimulation of acupuncture points, and advantages to apply on needle-forbidden acupuncture points, such as on umbilicus where regulates effect on fat metabolism through influencing blood circulation in abdominal area. Many healthy adults use the efficacy of laser acupuncture for fat deduction and reduce waist circumference for purpose to lose weight.

Section 6 Results of this study
本研究結果

The result shows that the comparison of the patient's effectiveness in the two groups between electro-acupuncture combined with laser and electro-acupuncture. Total efficiency rate was 90.00% which indicated significant result with electro-acupuncture combined with laser treatment, and the difference was highly significant at P<0.01. Thus, for treating simple obesity method was most effective by electro-acupuncture combined with laser. The results of the two groups of before and after treatment such as body weight, body fat rate (FAT) was decreased and changed significantly, and the difference was significant at P<0.05. Waist circumference and VFA decreased and significant difference was significant at P<0.01. BMI, hip and thigh circumference were decreased difference, but there were not shown statistically significance. It was shown apparently that the effect of electro-acupuncture combined with laser in reducing body fat rate, waist circumference and visceral fat was better than the electro-acupuncture group. By analyzing the results, it was shown that electro-acupuncture combined with laser treatment could further improve the efficacy of acupuncture treatment of simple obesity, especially the improvement of reducing body weight, waist circumference, body fat rate (FAT) and VFA which showed to be proved.

That indicates that electro-acupuncture combined with laser is able to treat even high level of VFA, risk of visceral, severe abdominal fat obesity, and this method is much better than electro-acupuncture treatment.

It is worth worthy, and it is necessary important clinical application for treating simple obesity by electro-acupuncture combined with laser.

6-1 Visceral fat and risk

Obesity, specially, visceral obesity is a global extensive known to be related to numerous pathological conditions, including metabolic syndrome, diabetes, hypertension, and cardiovascular disease. Several studies have shown that obesity increases visceral fat mass which is tightly linked to glucose intolerance, hyperinsulinemia, hypertriglyceridemia and metabolic syndrome. (49) When visceral adiposity increases, it caused risk of impaired glucose tolerance (IGT) independent of other adipose depots, insulin resistance, and insulin secretion. Body fat distribution is an important role in insulin syndrome. In particular, visceral adiposity is the key to the disease's insulin resistance, hyperinsulinemia, dyslipidemia, glucose intolerance and hypertension. (20) Thus, visceral fat is important role in the development to diabetes II. Impaired glucose tolerance is a strong predictor of diabetes II, cardiovascular and diabetes complications.

The International Diabetes Federation (IDF) convened a workshop held in May 2004 in London, UK, and participants included as well as from the World Health Organization (WHO) and National Cholesterol Education program. It was emphasized adiposity was the type most often associated with the metabolic abnormalities seen with diabetes and cardiovascular disease.

Simple Obesity is caused by fat metabolism disorder due to gene coding and endocrine dysfunction of compound of Lepton. The fat abdomen and the weight of Liver are influenced by high fat diet. Fat distribution of the ratio of waist circumference to hip circumference is an important prognostic indicator of the occurrence of metabolic abnormalities, diabetes II, hypertension, cardiovascular, stroke, and death which depends on the increased accumulation of intra-abdominal fat. These circumference ratios were relating to the amount of intra-abdominal fat and intra-abdominal fat ratio to subcutaneous abdominal fat.

Subcutaneous fat is less responsive than omental-adipose tissue to the lipolytic effects of epinephrine and norepinephrine and to the antilipolytic effect of insulin. Long-term exposure of the liver to high concentrations of fatty acids results in metabolic disorder.

By CT scanning of fat distribution, the fat accumulation of visceral fat obesity is more predominant in the intra-abdominal cavity than subcutaneous fat obesity. The Intra-abdominal cavity is accompanied by disorders of glucose and lipid metabolism and hypertension. It showed 90% of obese patients with ischemic heart disease were caused from visceral fat accumulation. For clinical and basic experiments, it is to be considered aging, imbalance of hormone, overintaking of sucrose and lack of physical exercise. Since intra-abdominal fat accumulation induces a high content of free fatty acids which goes into the Liver directly.

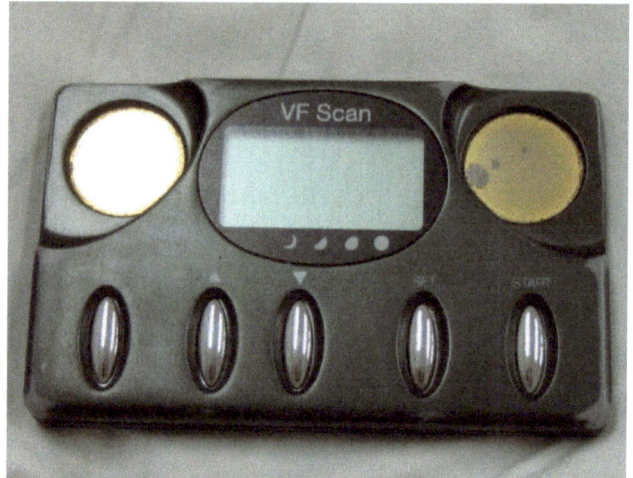
Visceral Fat Scan

6-2 Obesity Treatment and prospects

It has significant effects in obesity by physical training of high intensity exercise, such as cycling and jogging etc. as to refer to the earlier stated and demonstrated figure in activity Pyramid, page 24. It was reported that diet plus exercise such as walking 3-4 times a day was significantly effective weight-loss. Walking, this can be in safe performed and easiest way. To evaluate the effects of walking combined with diet therapy is 1000-1600 kcal/day. Walking should be at least 10,000 steps per day in daily routine. The studies were shown that simple obese person reduced the index of weight, waist circumference, ratio of waist circumference, buttocks and changed posture and plasma lipids, but also for improvement of insulin sensitivity by exercise.

Electro-acupuncture combined with laser treatment, diet therapy and exercise prescription including walking in 10,000 steps in routine every day should be effect on reducing Simple Obesity.

6-3 Discussion and experience

Obesity is a common and ancient group of metabolic syndromes. When the intaken calories are more than that of consumed, the extra calories are stored in the body in the form of fat. Obesity will be gradually developed when it is more than the physiological requirement and reached a certain level. So far, the etiology and pathogenesis of simple obesity is not yet very clear. From the perspective of traditional Chinese medicine, it belongs to the following aspects: irregular diet, lack of exercise, emotional disorders, senility, weakness due to chronic disease; Modern medicine believes it mainly includes genetic factors, psychological factors, endocrine factors, lifestyle and diet habit, etc.

The understanding of obesity from TCM has already been recorded as early as in Huangdi Neijing. "Their shoulders and armpit are usually broad, their muscles are thin, and skin is thick and black, their lips are plump and thick, their blood is blackish and turbid, the Qi in their body is unsmooth and slow in flowing. These kinds of people tend to keep forging ahead and are also generous to others." The greasy type is characterized by superabundance of Qi and looseness of skin. That is why their abdominal muscles are loose and their belly is hanging down. The muscular type is characterized by large capacity of the body. The greasy type is characterized by small body...So a person of greasy type is marked by loose abdominal muscles and hanging belly; a person of muscular type is marked by large capacity of both the upper and lower parts of the body; a person of fat type is marked by excessive fat and small body." (Spiritual Pivot) It is the earliest record about obesity classification. TCM believed that obesity was mainly caused by inner accumulation of fat and phlegm-dampness due to failing to transport and transform cereal essence of the spleen and stomach. It is said by Li Dongyuan that "When both the spleen and the stomach function properly, one will be strong and with good appetite. While both the spleen and stomach are in dysfunction, one will be skinny and with no appetite, or eat less but fat with weak limbs."

That is why the therapeutic principle is invigorating the spleen to resolve phlegm, eliminate fat and descend the turbid. Acupoints of the spleen meridian and the stomach meridian are commonly applied because disorders of the large and small intestines can be attributed to the stomach.

Apply ST25 (天俞 Tianshu) to dredge and coordinate the intestines, regulate Qi and promote bowel movements, ST36 (足三里 Zusanli) to suppress appetite and Ren12 (中脘 Zhongwan) to invigorate the spleen and the stomach, regulate the flow of Qi, ascend lucidity and descend turbidity in combination of SP6 (三阴交 Sanyinjiao) to promote transportation and transformation of the spleen and the stomach, eliminate turbid dampness, regulate menstruation and warm the lower part, SP10 (血海 Xuehai) to activate blood circulation, Ren6 (气海 Qihai) to regulate and tonify Qi, Ren9 (水分 Shuifen) to strengthen the spleen and the stomach and eliminate dampness, KI3 (太溪 Taixi) to tonify kidney Qi, clear away deficiency-heat, Liv3 (太冲 Taichong) to soothe the liver and regulate Qi and ST44 (内庭 Neiting) to clear away stomach-fire and dredge intestines. The joint application of all these acupoints is to coordinate the stomach and the intestines, suppress appetite and promote metabolism.

It is generally believed that high-frequency condensation wave is frequently used to relieve pain, tranquilize mind and ease muscle and vessel spasm by relaxing the nerve system; the use of low-frequency rarefaction wave is to evoke contraction and increase muscle and ligament tension; the use of condensation-rarefaction wave is to promote metabolism and Qi and blood circulation, increase nutrition of the tissues and alleviate inflammatory edema. It was reported in literature that frequency of 2Hz was more effective than that of 100Hz. It has been proved that frequency of 2Hz is effective to reduce weight while frequency of 100Hz to lower blood fat. So, it is worth experimenting with 2/100Hz alternating mode to supplement each method. This research applied condensation-rarefaction wave electrical stimulation on the abdominal acupoints to strengthen needling sensation and obtain continuous stimulation thus promoting gastrointestinal peristalsis and fat metabolism.

1 Effects of electro-acupuncture

Electro-acupuncture (EA) combining traditional acupuncture and modern science has been widely applied and achieved affirmative effects clinically.

high-frequency condensation wave is frequently used to relieve pain, tranquilize mind and ease muscle and vessel spasm by relaxing the nerve system; the use of low-frequency rarefaction wave is to evoke contraction and increase muscle and ligament tension; the use of condensation-rarefaction wave is to promote metabolism and Qi and blood circulation, increase nutrition of the tissues and alleviate inflammatory edema. Most patients of simple obesity with thick abdominal fat are poorly sensitive to acupuncture. EA can strengthen the needling sensation. By using alternative mode of three frequencies, we obtain continuous stimulation on the abdominal acupoints and avoid tolerance thus promoting gastrointestinal peristalsis and fat metabolism; so that more fat can be used for energy-supply and weight loss can be achieved. This method is significantly effective in central obese patients with large waist circumference.

2 Effects of laser acupuncture

Compared with traditional acupuncture treatment, the laser acupuncture advanced in being safe without damage, no broken needle during treatment and aseptic manipulation, causing patients no pain and fainting and also it is easy to manipulate. Both methods work on the body through the meridians and collaterals.

During treatment, within the patients' tolerance, we applied low power output laser on REN 8 (神阙 Shenque), the liver region and local parts of high-ratio body fat on condensation-rarefaction wave at the wavelength of 650nm and under the laser output power of 5mw. By doing this, not only can the stomach and intestines be coordinated but also the special penetrating power of laser can work on deeper subcutaneous tissues influencing penetrability of cell membrane and activity of enzymes, thus promoting body metabolism and stimulating blood circulation by causing blood vessels in deep tissues to dilate, which will accelerate decomposition of fat and reduce subcutaneous fat and visceral fat as well. So, in this research, we found that laser-electro acupuncture can achieve a better result in reducing FAT, VFA and waist circumference than electro-acupuncture.

3. Conclusion

By combined with the theory of TCM (traditional Chinese medicine) and modern research of simple obesity patients with visceral fat, efficacy of comparison between electro-acupuncture alone and electro-acupuncture with laser treatment are;

(1) Electro-acupuncture and electro-acupuncture combined with laser treatment of simple obesity is the most effective way to lose weight which is non-toxific, simple method, no side-effects, safe, most effective therapy, reliable and inexpensive.

(2) Pathogenesis obesity is generally relating visceral reasons which are dampness, phlegm, Spleen, liver Qi stagnation, kidney metabolism and stomach heat, Yin and Yang, Qi and Blood disorders.

(3) Electro-acupuncture combined with laser treatment for simple obesity for reducing waist circumference, visceral fat, BMI and fat rate is better method more than electro-acupuncture alone treatment.

Section 7 Weight Loss by Acpuncture treatment 减肥针炎

7.1 Obesity

Obesity relates to overeating (Diet), and function of Stomach and Sprain.

Obesity often causes Stroke and Diabetes.

Obesity is caused by overeating, indulge food, emotional, cream fat accumulation in Stomach, Sprain and Phlegm.

Liv + KI Qi go down, and Ki Qi and SP function inferred.

Result-Pathogenic
1. Liv-Qi stagnation + ST (digest) +SP channel cause to Phlegm
2. Phlegm + Damp
3. Status: Heat

Treatment method

As it becomes excessive ST and then SP will be weak. Therefore, reduce ST channel and tonify Spleen. (ST channel (Foot) use.

(1) Standard weight: Calculates for
Standard weight: (height-100) x 0.9

(2) BMI (Body Mass Index): Calculates for obesity degree.
(kg/m^2) Body weight/height^2

(3) BMI degree
- Mild: 25-30 %
- Medium: 30-40 %
- Severe: more than 40 %

7.1.1 Method for Measurement
- When patient gets measurement, it must be used the same scale.
- Patient must use the same cloth when he/she gets the measurement.
- It can be taken one course will be 15 treatments.
- Patient must be relaxed to take measurement.
- Patient must take off cloth.
- Clinic must use the tape for measurement.
- Chest measurement: on nipple.
- Waist measurement: on navel.
- Hip line: measure most high line.
- Measure Groin
- Measure Calf
- Measure Arm line: meets L.I.11 (曲池)
- Write clinical record.
- Take a look for comparison of "before and present"

- Write complication on record.

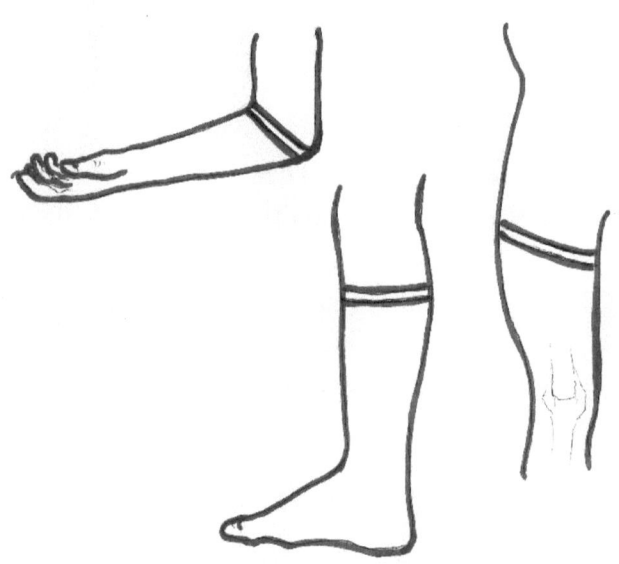

Measure arm and leg line

7.1.2 Connection Channel for Weight Loss

(1) ST channel, SP channel, BL channel and Ren channel.

(2) Add point: Yin Heel channel and Yang Heel channel.

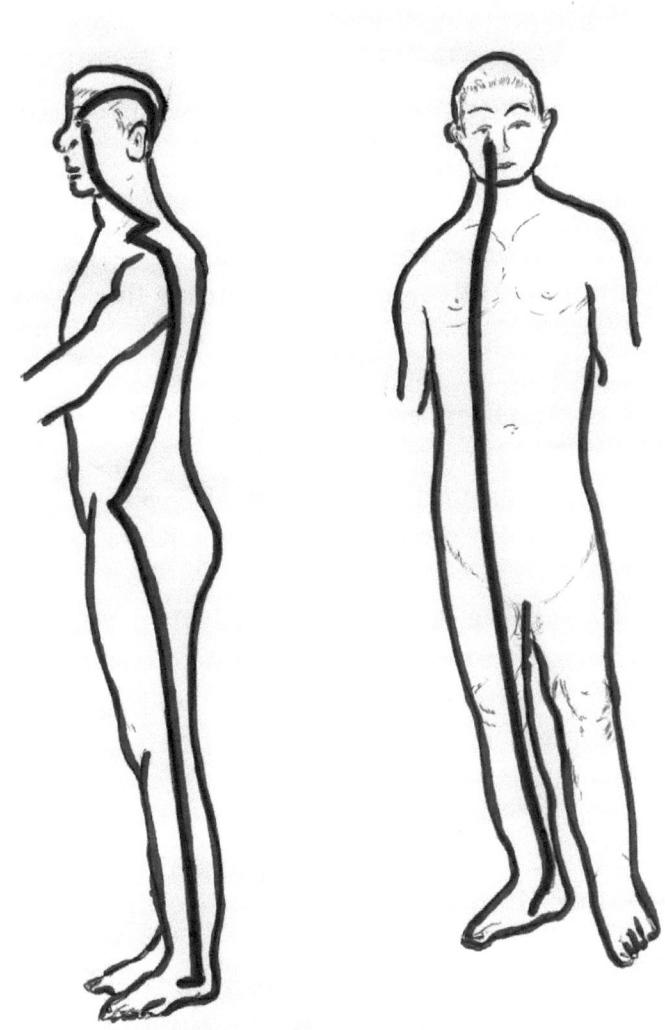

The Yang Heel channel   The Yin Heel channel

- Yin heel channel starts from KI 6 (照海).
- Yang heel channel starts from BL 62 (申脈).

7.1.3 Syndrome

Obesity generally speaking includes five syndromes.

1. Excessive Heat in ST and LI
2. Dampness due to SP deficiency
3. Qi stagnation of Liv
4. Yang deficiency of SP + KI
5. Yin deficiency of Liv + KI

1. Excessive Heat in ST and LI

Manifestation: heavy, big/excessive appetite, diet is sweet, fatty, greasy, salty, fried, lot of water (cold). dislike heat, dry stool, constipation.

Tongue: red, yellow coating

Pulse: wiry, slippery, rapid.

More than 80 % of patient are this type.

2. Dampness due to SP deficiency

Accumulating phlegm, SP function is not good (transport food+water), poor appetite, lassitude

(Qi+loss of blood), heaviness due to dampness, abdorminal distention, loose stool (contains water), scanty urine, edema in limbs (some cases).
Tongue body: pale colour, enlarge (swollen) and tender.
Tongue coating: thin, greasy and various colour.
Pulse: deep, thread (thin) slippery pulse.

3. Qi stagnation of LIV
Heavy body, distension, fullness of hypochondriac region, emotional problem depression, irritability, insomnia.
Menstruation: irregular cycle, alternated cycle, longer, shorter and no menstruation, amenorrhea colour is fresh red, thickness, sticky, clots.
Tongue coating: white, thin and greasy coating.
Pulse: thread, wildly.

4. Yang deficiency of SP+KI
Heavy body, KI deficiency, Lumber soreness, Yang Qi and Yin Qi deficiency, SP Yang deficiency (lassitude, weakness, no energy), cold, aversion to cold limb, facial puffiness, loose stool, abdominal distension, impotent, cold uterus

Tongue coating: pale, thin greasy, large (swollen)

Pulse: deep, thready, weak.

5. **Yin deficiency of Liv and KI**

Heavy body, dizziness (head), blurred vision, distending headache, Lumber soreness from KI deficiency, hot sensation from Yin deficiency, low fever in the afternoon.

Tongue: flat red (tip red) (indicate heat), dry without moisture

Puls: thready, thin, rapid (sign of heat inside of body), slightly wiry.

7.1.4 Channel point for Treatment

Obesity general speaking is four channels selected which are:

- ST channel
- SP (leg) channel
- Ren channel
- BL channel

Selection point:

1. Syndrome selection
2. Choose point along channel from four.
3. Choose point according to symptom.

4. Choose local/regional point.

Essential point:

- Ren 12 (中脘 Zhongwan)
- ST 25 (天枢 Tianshu)
- Ren 9 (水分 Shuifen)
- ST36 (足三里 Zusanli)
- SP 6 (三阴交 Sanyinjiao)
- ST 37 (上巨虚 Shangjuxu)

ST 37 (上巨虚 Shangjuxu) is lower He-sea point of Large Intestine, and the point of Sea of Blood.

7.2 Patient Syndrome Pattern

As it has described earlier, there are five patterns.

1. Eliminate Heat, promote ST+LI
2. Dampness SP deficiency
3. Qi Liv stagnation
4. Yang deficiency SP+KI
5. Yin deficiency

1. Eliminate Heat, promote ST+LI

- LI-11 (曲池 Quchi)
- LI-4 (合谷 Hegu)
- ST-21 (梁门 Liangmen)
- ST-44 (内庭 Neiting)

ST21(梁门 Liangmen) is an important point of digestion. ST-44 (内庭 Neiting) is the water point of Stomach channel, eliminate heat and restricting appetizer. Clear heat and promote digestion.

2. Dampness SP deficiency
- ST-40 (豐隆 Fenglong)
- SP-9 (陰陵泉 Yinglingquan)
- Ren-6 (气海 Qihai)
- ST-29 (帰来 Guilai)

SP-9 (陰陵泉 Yinglingquan) can tonify damp. ST-29 (帰来 Guilai) can regulate menstruation.

3. Qi Liv stagnation
- BL-18 (肝俞 Ganshu)
- Liv-2 (行间 Xingjian)
- Liv-3 (太冲 Taichong)
- GB-34 (陽陵泉 Yanglingquan)

These four points can reduce fire and heat. GB-34 (陽陵泉 Yanglingquan) is the He-sea point of Gall

Bladder and can cure disorder of sinew and clears Liv Qi.

4. Yang deficiency SP+KI

- BL-20 (脾俞 Pishu)
- BL-23 (肾俞 Senshu)
- Ren-4 (關元 Guanyuan)
- SP-9 (陰陵泉 Yinglingquan)

Ren-4 (關元 Guanyuan) is Front MU point of Small Intestine, and meeting point of Conception channel with SP, Liv, and KI.

5. Yin deficiency

- BL-18 (肝俞 Ganshu)
- BL-23 (肾俞 Senshu)
- KI-3 (太溪 Taixi)
- KI-6 (照海 Zhaohai)

KI-3 (太溪 Taixi) is Yuan source of Kidney channel.

7.2.1 Patient Severe Syndrome

1. Constipation
2. Sleepness
3. Abdorminal distention
4. Shortness of breath and palpitation

1. Constipation
- SJ-6 (支溝 Zhigou)
- ST-39 (下巨虛 Xiajyushu)
- KI-6 (照海 Zhaohai)
- BL-57(承山 Chengshan)

SJ-6 (支溝 Zhigou) can help to move stool. ST-39 (下巨虛 Xiajyushu) is Lower He-Sea point of Small Intestine and point of Sea of Blood. As Yin deficiency, stool become dry, this point will help to supply water to push boat. BL-57(承山 Chengshan) is constipation point and helps bowel movement.

2. Sleepness
- KI-6 (照海 Zhaohai)
- BL-62 (申脈 Shenmai)

Too much Yin than Yang. KI-6 (照海 Zhaohai) can reduce Yin, and BL-62 (申脈 Shenmai) can tonify Yang.

3. Abdorminal distention
- BL-27 (小腸俞 Xiaochangshu)
- ST-39 (下巨俞 Xiajushu)

BL-27 (小肠俞 Xiaochangshu) is Back shu point of Small Intestine and ST-39 (下巨俞 Xiajushu) is Lower He-sea point of Small Intestine.

4. Shortness of breath and palpitation
- HT-7 (神门 Shenmen)
- P-6 (内關 Neiguan)

References 参考文献

1. Yung-Ting Chuang, Tzong-Shiun Li, Tze-Yi Lin, Chih-Jung Hsu1. An unusual complication related to acupuncture point catgut embedding treatment of obesity, Acupunct Med December 2011; Vol 29 No 4

2. Wen-Long Hu, Chih-Hao Chang, Yu-Chiang Hung. Clinical observations on laser acupuncture in simple obesity, Diabetes, Obesity and Metabolism, Blackwell Publishing Ltd, 12: 2010; 553–554.

3. G. Litscher. The application of bioengineering of acupuncture to the treatment of diabetes, insulin resistance and obesity. 2010; 12: 553–554

4. Jingke Guo, Yue Chen, Bin Yuan, Shutao Liu, Pingfan Rao. Effects of Intracellular Superoxide Removal at Acupoints with TAT-SOD on Obesity, Free Radical Biology & Medicine, 51, 2011; 2185–2189

5. Y. Sui, H. L. Zhao, V. C. W. Wong, N. Brown, X. L. Li, A. K. L. Kwan, H. L. W. Hui, E. T. C. Ziea and J. C. N. Chan. A systematic review on use

of Chinese medicine and acupuncture for treatment of obesity. Obesity Reviews, 2012

6.   Fei Wanga, De Run Tiana,b,, Patrick Tsoc, Ji Sheng Hana. Arcuate nucleus of hypothalamus is involved in mediating the satiety effect of electroacupuncture in obese rats, Peptides 32 (2011) 2394–2399

7.   Japan Society for the Study of Obesity. New Criteria for "Obesity Disease" in Japan, Circulation Journal 2002; 66: 987 –992

8.   Naoko Horie, Hideaki Komiya, Yutaka Mori and Naoko Tajima. New Body Mass Index Criteria of Central Obesity for Male Japanese, Tohoku J. Exp. Med., 2006; 208,83-86

10.   JM Lacey, AM Tershakovec and GD Foster. Acupuncture for the treatment of obesity: A review of the Evidence, Nature Publishing Group, International Journal of Obesity 2003; 27, 419–427

11.   Rita Romani, Gianna Evelina De Medio, Simona di Tullio,Rosa Lapalombella, Irene Pirisinu, Vittoria Margonato, Arsenio Veicsteinas, Marina Marini, and Gabriella Rosi. Modulation of paraoxonase 1 and 3 expression after moderate exercise training in the rat, the American Society for

Biochemistry and Molecular Biology, Inc. Journal of Lipid Research, 2009; Vol. 50

12.   Takayoshi Suganami, Junko Nishida, Yoshihiro Ogawa. A Paracrine Loop Between Adipocytes and Macrophages Aggravates Inflammatory Changes Role of Free Fatty Acids and Tumor Necrosis Factor, Journal of American Heart Association, Arterioscler Thromb Vasc Biol 2005; 25: 2062-2068

13.   Jean-Pierre Despre, Isabelle Lemieux, Jean Bergeron, Philippe Pibarot, Patrick Mathieu, Eric Larose, Josep Rode´s-Cabau, Olivier F. Bertrand, Paul Poirier. Abdominal Obesity and the Metabolic Syndrome: Contribution to Global Cardiometabolic Risk, Journal of American Heart Association, Arterioscler Thrombosis, Vascular Biology, 2008; 28:1039-1049

14.   Satya P. Kalra. Appetite and Body Weight Regulation: Minireview Is It All in the Brain, Neuron, 1997; Vol. 19, 227–230

15.   George A Bray and Barry M Popkin. Dietary fat intake does affect obesity, American Society for Clinical Nutrition, 1998; 68: 1157–73

16.   Kristina M. Utzschneider, Darcy B. Carr, Rebecca L. Hull, Keiichi Kodama, Jane B. Shofer,

Barbara M. Retzlaff, Robert H. Knopp, and Steven E. Kahn1. Impact of Intra-Abdominal Fat and Age on Insulin Sensitivity and BCell Function, American Diabetes Association Diabetes, 2004, VOL.53

17.   Satoshi Nishimura, Ichiro Manabe, Mika Nagasaki, Kinya Seo, Hiroshi Yamashita, Yumiko Hosoya, Mitsuru Ohsugi, Kazuyuki Tobe, Takashi Kadowaki, Ryozo Nagai, and Seiryo Sugiura. In vivo imaging in mice reveals local cell dynamics and inflammation in obese adipose tissue, The Journal of Clinical Investigation, Research article, 2008; Vol. 118, 2.

18.   Fida A Bacha, Rola Saad, Neslihan Gungor, Janine Janosky, and Silva A Arslanian. Obesity, Regional Fat Distribution, and Syndrome X in Obese Black Versus White Adolescents: Race Differential in Diabetogenic and Atherogenic Risk Factors, The Journal of Clinical Endocrinology & Metabolism, The Endocrine Society, 2003; 88(6): 2534–2540

19.   Bernardo Lernardo Leo Wajchenberg. Subcutaneous and Visceral Adipose Tissue: Their Relation to the Metabolic Syndrome, Endocrine Reviews,The Endocrine Society, 2000; 21(6): 697–738

20. Tomoshige Hayashi, Edward J Boyko. Donna L Leonetti, Marguerite J. Mcneely, Laura Newell-Morris, Steven E. Kahn, Wilfred Y Fujimoto. Visceral Adiposity and the Risk of Impaired Glucose Tolerance, Epidemiology Health Services Psychosocial Research, Diabetes Care, 2003; Vol. 26, 3

21. Tomoshige Hayashi, Edward J. Boyko. Donna L. Leonetti, Marguerite J. McNeely, Laura Newell-Morris, Steven E. Kahn, and Wilfred Y. Fujimoto. Visceral Adiposity Is an Independent Predictor of Incident Hypertension in Japanese Americans, Ann Intern Med. 2004; 140, 992-1000.

22. Jennifer L. Kuk, Peter T. Katzmarzyk. Milton Z. Nichaman, Timothy S. Church, Steven N. Blair, and Robert Ross, Visceral Fat is an Independent Predictor of All-cause Mortality in Men, Obesity, 2006; Vol. 14, 2

23. M Labib. The investigation and management of obesity, J Clin Pathol, 2003; 56: 17-25

24. lHj Bourne. Economic Aspects of Tender Spot Injection Therapy, Acupuncture Med; 1996; 14,116-120

25.   Mini P. Sajan, Mary L. Standaert, Sonali Nimal, Usha Varanasi,Tina Pastoor, Stephen Mastorides, Ursula Braun, Michael Leitges, and Robert V. Farese1. The critical role of atypical protein kinase C in activating hepatic SREBP-1c and NFkB in obesity, Journal of Lipid Research, 2009; Vol.50

26.   A Apostolopoulos, M Karavis. Overeating: Treatment of Obesity and Anxiety by Auricular Acupuncture, an Analysis of 800 cases, Acupunct Med; 1996; 14, 116-1

27.   Takemasa Shiraishi, Mariko Onoe, Taka-Aki Kojima, Teruo Kageyama, Shoichi Sawatsugawa, Kohji Sakurai, Hironobu Yoshimatsu and Toshiie Sakata. Effects of Bilateral Auricular Acupuncture Stimulation on Body Weight in Healthy Volunteers and Mildly Obese Patients, Experimental Biology and Medicine 2003; 228:1201-1207

28.   Martin S. Mok, Lawrence N. Parker, Sandra Voina, and George A Bray. Treatment of Obesity by Acupuncture, The American Journal of Clinical Nutrition 29, 1976; 832-835

29.   Tuomo Rankinen, Aamir Zuberi, Yvon C. Chagnon, S. John Weisnagel,George Argyropoulos,Brandon Walts, Louis Pe´russe, and

Claude Bouchard. The Human Obesity Gene Map: The 2005 Update Obesity, 2006; Vol. 14, No. 4

31.   F Contaldo, M Mancini and L A Reed. Liver and Obesity, Gut, 1985; 26, 1096

32.   Luigie.Adinolfi, Michele Gambardella, Augusto Andreana, Marie-franc, Oise Tripodi, Riccardo Utili, and Giuseppe Ruggiero. Steatosis Accelerates the Progression of Liver Damage of Chronic Hepatitis C Patients and Correlates with Specific HCV Genotype and Visceral Obesity, the American Association for the Study of Liver Diseases, Hepatology, 2001; Vol. 33, 6

33.   Ryo Suzuki, Kazuyuki Tobe, Masashi Aoyama, Atsushi Inoue, Kentaro Sakamoto, Toshimasa Yamauchi, Junji Kamon, Naoto Kubota, Yasuo Terauchi,Hironobu Yoshimatsu, Munehide Matsuhisa, Shoichiro Nagasaka, Hitomi Ogata,Kumpei Tokuyama, Ryozo Nagai, and Takashi Kadowaki. Both Insulin Signaling Defects in the Liver and Obesity Contribute to Insulin Resistance and Cause Diabetes in Irs2 Mice, The Journal of Biological Chemistry, The American Society for Biochemistry and Molecular Biology, Inc. 2004; Vol. 279, 24, 25039–25049

34. A. Colin Bell, Keyou Ge, and Barry M. Popkin. the Road to Obesity or the Path to Prevention: Motorized Transportation and Obesity in China, Obesity Research, 2002; Vol. 10, 4

35. Parvez Hossain, Bisher Kawar, and Meguid El Nahas. Obesity and Diabetes in the Developing World – A Growing Challenge, The New England Journal of Medicine, 2007; 356; 3

36. Bin Xui, Zen-Pin Lin, Ling-Ling Wang, Lawrence W. Lan, Jaung-Geng Lin, Tsung-Jung Ho. Effects of Electroacupuncture on Obese rats' weight reduction, School of Chinese Medicine, College of Chinese Medicine, China Medical University, Taiwan

37. Tsutomu Shimada, Tomoko Akase, Mitsutaka Kosugi, and Masaki Aburada. Preventive Effect of Boiogito on Metabolic Disorders in the TSOD Mouse, a Model of Spontaneous Obese Type II Diabetes Mellitus, Hindawi Publishing Corporation, Evidence-Based Complementary and Alternative Medicine, 2011, ID 93173, 1-8

38. Jun-ichi Yamakawa, Junji Moriya, Takashi Takahashi, Atsushi Ishige, Yoshiharu Motoo, Fumihiko Yoshizaki and Tsugiyasu Kanda. A Kampo Medicine, Boi-ogi-to, Inhibits Obesity in Ovariectomized Rats, CAM 2010; 7(1)87–95

39. Mehmet Tuğrul Cabıoğlu, Neyhan Ergene. Changes in Serum Leptin and Beta Endorphin Levels with Weight Loss by Electroacupuncture and Diet Restriction in Obesity Treatment, The American Journal of Chinese Medicine, 2006; Vol. 34, No. 1, 1–11

40. Takemasa Shiraishi, Mariko Onoe, Takaaki Kojima, Teruo Kageyama, Shoichi Sawatsugawa, Kohji Sakurai, Hironobu Yoshimatsu, and Toshie Sakata. Effects of Bilateral Auricular Acupuncture Stimulation on Body Weight in Healthy Volunteers and Mildly Obese Patients, Experimental Biology and Medicine 2003; 228:1201-1207

41. Chizuko Hioki and Makoto Arai. Bofutsushosan use for Obesity with IGT: search for scientific basis and development of effective therapy with Kampo medicine, J. Trad. Med., 2007; 24, 115-127

42. C-H Hsu, K-C Hwang, C-L Chao, J-G Lin, S-T Kao and P Chou. Effects of electroacupuncture in reducing weight and waist circumference in obese women: a randomized, International Journal of Obesity 2005; 29, 1379–1384

43. Xiao-Guang Liu, Juan Zhang, Jian-Liang Lu, Timon Cheng-Yi Liu. Laser Acupuncture

Reduces Body Fat in Obese Female Undergraduate Students, the Science and Technology Planning Foundation of Guangdong Province, China (2011B031600006) and National Natural Science Laboratory of Laser Sports Medicine, South China Normal University, Guangzhou

44. Wei Shougang and Xie Xincai. Acupuncture for the Treatment of Simple Obesity: Basic and Clinical Aspects, Beijing Natural Science Foundation (No. 7112014), Capital Medical University, China

45. Huijuan Cao, Mei Han, Xun Li, Shangjuan Dong, Yongmei Shang, Qian Wang, Shu Xu, Jianping Liu. Clinical research evidence of cupping therapy in China: a systematic literature review, BMC Complementary and Alternative Medicine, 2010; 10:70

46. Mei Chen, Shi Xiaoyang, Xu Bin, Guyi Huang, Dong Qin, Xu Lanfeng , Li Kaiping Zhang Jianbin, Mu Yanyun. Clinical observation of acupuncture therapy of simple obesity, Clinical Study of Treating Simple Obesity with Acupotomy, Chinese Acupuncture 2011; 31 (6) 539-542

47.   Issues for DSM-V: Should Obesity Be Included as a Brain Disorder? Am J Psychiatry 2007; 164:5

48.   Is Obesity a Mental Health Issue? MediLexicon International Ltd., 2004

49.   Britt G. Gabrielsson, Jenny M. Johansson, Malin Lo"nn, Margareta Jernås,Torsten Olbers,Markku Peltonen, Ingrid Larsson,Lars Lo"nn, Lars Sjo"stro"m, Bjo"rn Carlsson,and Lena M.S. Carlsson. High Expression of Complement Components in Omental Adipose Tissue in Obese Men, Obesity Research, 2003; Vol. 11 No.6

50.   Schwartz, Michael W.; Woods, Stephen C; Porte, Daniel Jr; Seeley, Randy J.; Baskin, Denis G. Central nervous system control of food intake, Ovid: Schwartz: Nature, Volume 404(6778), 2000; 661-671

51.   Daniel Porte, Denis G. Baskin, and Michael W. Schwartz. Leptin and Insulin Action in the Central Nervous System, Nutrition Reviews, Vol. 60, No. 10, 2002; (II)S20–S29

53.   P. Pottie, N. Presle, B. Terlain, P. Netter, D. Mainard, F. Berenbaum. Obesity and osteoarthritis: more complex than predicted, Ann Rheum Dis 2006; 65:1403–1405

54.		Elena Losina, Rochelle P. Walensky, William M. Reichmann, Holly L. Holt, Hanna Gerlovin, Daniel H. Solomon, Joanne M. Jordan,David J. Hunter, Lisa G. Suter, Alexander M. Weinstein, A. David Paltiel, and Jeffrey N. Katz. Impact of Obesity and Knee Osteoarthritis on Morbidity and Mortality in Older Americans, Ann Intern Med. 2011;154:217-226

55.		Natalia Danilovich, P. Sureshbabu, Weirong Xing, Maria Gerdes, Hanumanthappa Krishnamurthy and M. Ramam Sairam, Estrogen Eficiency. Obesity, and Skeletal Abnormalities in Follicle-Stimulating Hormone Receptor Knockout (FORKO) Female Mice, The Endocrine Society, Endo 2000; Vol. 141, 11

56.		Christopher L. Amling, Robert H. Riffenburgh, Leon Sun, Judd W. Moul, Raymond S. Lance,Leo Kusuda, Wade J. Sexton, Douglas W. Soderdahl, Timothy F. Donahue, John P. Foley,Andrew K. Chung, and David G. McLeod. Pathologic Variables and Recurrence Rates as Related to Obesity and Race in Men with Prostate Cancer Undergoing Radical Prostatectomy, Journal of Clinical Oncology, 2004; Vol. 22, 3

57.		Qian Gao, Michael J. Wolfgang, Susanne Neschen, Katsutaro Morino, Tamas L. Horvath,

Gerald I. Shulman, and Xin-Yuan Fu. Disruption of neural signal transducer and activator of transcription 3 causes obesity, diabetes, infertility, and thermal dysregulation, The National Academy of Sciences of the USA, 2004; vol. 101,13, 4661–4666

58.   Meir J Stampfer, K Malcolm Malclure, Graham A Colditz, JoAnn E Manson, and Walter C Willette. Risk of Symptomatic Gallstones in Women with Severe Obesity, Am J Clin Nutr 1992; 55:652-8

59.   Song-Hae Bok, Myung-Hee Kim, Eun Eai Kim, Mung-Sook Chok, Surk-Sik Moon, Kyu-Tae Chang. Powder or extracts of plant leaves with anti-obesity effects and anti-obesity food comprising them, United States Patent Application Publication, US 2005/0003026 A, 2005

60.   Xu Bin and Liu Zhi-chen. Chinese-English Edition of Acupuncture for Weight Loss, Shanghai Scientific and Technical Publishers, 2007

61.   Ai Bing-Wei, Wang Qi-Cai. Acupuncture and Moxibution for Obesity, 2010, ISBN 978-7-117-13340-1

62.   JG Karam, SI McFarlane. Diabetes, Metabolic Syndrome and Obesity: Targets and Therapy, Dove Press journal: 2010; 3 95–112

63. George Binh Lenon, Kang Xiao Li, Yung-Hsien Chang, AngelaWeihong Yang, Clifford Da Costa, Chun Guang Li, Marc Cohen, NeilMann, and Charlie C. L. Xue. Efficacy and Safety of a Chinese Herbal Medicine Formula (RCM-104) in theManagement of Simple Obesity: A Randomized, Placebo-Controlled Clinical Trial, Hindawi Publishing Corporation, Evidence-Based Complementary and Alternative Medicine, 2012; Article ID 435702, 11 pages

64. Li-Wei Chien, Miao-Hsiang Lin, Hsueh-Yu Chung, and Chi-Feng Liu. Transcutaneous Electrical Stimulation of Acupoints Changes Body Composition and Heart Rate Variability in PostmenopausalWomen with Obesity, Hindawi Publishing Corporation, Evidence-Based Complementary and Alternative Medicine 2011; Article ID 862121, 7 pages

65. Erin LeBlanc, Elizabeth O'Connor, Evelyn P. Whitlock, Carrie Patnode, Tanya Kapka. Screening for and Management of Obesity and Overweight in Adults, AHRQ Publication No. 11-05159-EF-1; 2011

66. Rong-Tsung Lin, Chung-Yuh Tzeng, Yu-Chen Lee, Wai-Jane Ho, Juei-Tang Cheng, Jaung-Geng Lin6 and Shih-Liang Chang. Acute effect of

electroacupuncture at the Zusanli acupoints on decreasing insulin resistance as shown by lowering plasma free fatty acid levels in steroid-background male rats, BMC Complementary and Alternative Medicine 2009; 9:26

67.   John Zhang, Nelson Marquina, George Oxinos, Amy Saud, Derek Ngd. Effect of laser acupoint treatment on blood pressure and body weight—a pilot study, Journal of Chiropractic Medicine, 2008; 7, 134–139

68.   Evrim B. Turkbey, Robyn L. McClelland, Richard A. Kronmal, Gregory L. Burke, Diane E. Bild, Russell P. Tracy, Andrew E. Arai, João A. C. Lima, and David A. Bluemke. The Impact of Obesity on the Left Ventricle: The Multi-Ethnic Study of Atherosclerosis (MESA), JACC Cardiovasc Imaging; 2010; 3(3): 266–274.

69.   Ahmed Elmarakby, and John D. Imig. Obesity is the Major Contributor to Vascular Dysfunction and Inflammation in High Fat Diet Hypertensive Rats, Clin Sci (Lond). 2010; 118(4): 291–301

70.   Emily L.Gilbert and Michael J. Ryan. High Dietary Fat Promotes Visceral Obesity and Impaired Endothelial Function in Female Mice with

Systemic Lupus Erythematosus, Gend Med. 2011; 8(2): 150–155

71.   Kazunari Kaneko, Takahisa Kimata, Shoji Tsuji, Kazumi Shiraishi, Kuniaki Yamauchi, Mutsumi Murakami, Teruo Kitagawa. Impact of obesity on childhood Kidney, Pediatric Reports 2011; vol. 3: e27

72.   Andrew S. Bomback Philip J. Klemmer. Interaction of Aldosterone and Extracellular Volume in the Pathogenesis of Obesity-Associated Kidney Disease: A Narrative Review, Am J Nephrol 2009;30, 140–146

73.   Nicole Vogelzangs, Stephen B Kritchevsky, Aartjan TF Beekman, Gretchen A Brenes, Anne B Newman, Suzanne Satterfield, Kristine Yaffe, Tamara B Harris, and Brenda WJH Penninx. Obesity and Onset of Significant Depressive symptoms: Results from a community-based cohort of older men and women, J Clin Psychiatry. 2010; 71(4): 391–399

74.   Pathmaja Paramsothy, Robert Knopp, Alain G. Bertoni, Michael Y. Tsai, Tessa Rue, and Susan R. Heckbert. Combined Hyperlipidemia in relation to Race/Ethnicity, Obesity, and Insulin Resistance in the Multi-Ethnic Study of

Atherosclerosis (MESA), Metabolism. 2009; 58(2): 212–219

75.   Taryn P Stewart, Hyoung Yon Kim, Arnold M Saxton, Jung Han Kim. Genetic and genomic analysis of hyperlipidemia, obesity and diabetes using (C57BL/6J TALLYHO/JngJ) F2 mice, Stewart et al. BMC Genomics 2010; 11:713

76.   Li Tang, Masaru Kubota, Ayako Nagai, Kimiyo Mamemoto, Masakuni Tokuda. Hyperuricemia in obese children and adolescents: the relationship with metabolic syndrome, Pediatric Reports 2010; Vol. 2: e12

77.   Tomoyuki Akiyama, Masato Yoneda, Masahiko Inamori, Hiroshi Iida, Hiroki Endo, Kunihiro Hosono, Kyoko Yoneda, Koji Fujita, Tomoko Koide, Chikako Tokoro, Hirokazu Takahashi, Ayumu Goto, Yasunobu Abe, Hiroyuki Kirikoshi, Noritoshi Kobayashi, Kensuke Kubota, Satoru Saito and Atsushi Nakajima. Visceral obesity and the risk of Barrett's esophagus in Japanese Patients with non-alcoholic fatty liver disease, BMC Gastroenterology 2009; 9:56

78.   SC Larsson,1 and A Wolk. Obesity and the risk of gallbladder cancer: a meta-analysis, British Journal of Cancer 2007; 96, 1457–1461

79.	Jean-Louis Frossard, Pierre Lescuyer, Catherine M Pastor. Experimental evidence of obesity as a risk factor for severe acute pancreatitis, World J Gastroenterol 2009; 15(42): 5260-5265

80.	Christopher Zammit, Helen Liddicoat, Ian Moonsie, Himender Makker. Obesity and respiratory diseases, International Journal of General Medicine 2010; 3 335–343

81.	Alan R. Schwartz, Susheel P. Patil, Samuel Squier, Hartmut Schneider, Jason P. Kirkness, and Philip L. Smith. Obesity and upper airway control during sleep, Appl Physiol. 2010; 108(2): 430–435

82.	Peter Mancuso. Obesity and lung inflammation, J Appl Physiol. 2010; 108(3): 722–728

83.	Antonios Stavropoulos-Kalinoglou, Giorgos S Metsios, Yiannis Koutedakis, Alan M Nevill, Karen M Douglas, Athanasios Jamurtas, Jet J C S Veldhuijzen van Zanten, Mourad Labib, and George D Kitas.	Redefining overweight and obesity in rheumatoid arthritis patients, Ann Rheum Dis 2007;66:1316–1321

84.	Luigi Manni, Thomas Lundeberg, Agneta Holmäng, Luigi Aloe and Elisabet Stener-Victorin. Effect of electro-acupuncture on ovarian expression

146

of (1)- and (2)-adrenoceptors, and p75 neurotrophin receptors in rats with steroid-induced polycystic ovaries, Reproductive Biology and Endocrinology 2005; 3:21

85.   Antonio Macciò and Clelia Madeddu. Obesity, Inflammation, and Postmenopausal Breast Cancer: Therapeutic   Implications, TheScientificWorld Journal, 2011; 11, 2020–2036

86.   Mattew W. Gillman, Helena Oakey, Peter A. Baghurst, Roberte E. Volkmer, Jeffrey S. Robinson Franzcog, Caroline A. Crowther Franzcog. Effect of Treatment of Gestational Diabetes Mellitus on Obesity in the Next Generation, Diabetes Care 2010; 33:964–968

87.   Suparna Rajan, Marguerite J. McNeely, Catherine Warms; Barry Goldstein. Clinical Assessment and Management of Obesity in Individuals with Spinal Cord Injury: A Review, J Spinal Cord Med. 2008; 31(4): 361–372

88.   Fengxia Liang, Rui Chen, Atsushi Nakagawa, Makoto Nishizawa, Shinichi Tsuda,Hua Wang, and Daisuke Koya. Low-Frequency Electroacupuncture Improves Insulin Sensitivity in Obese Diabetic Mice through Activation of SIRT1/PGC-1α in Skeletal Muscle, Evidence-Based

Complementary and Alternative Medicine, 2011; Article ID 735297, 9 pages

89.   Xavier Pi-Sunyer. The Medical Risks of Obesity, Postgrad Med., 2009; 121(6): 21–33

90.   Hamid Abdi, Baixiao Zhao, Mahsa Darbandi, Majid Ghayour-Mobarhan, Shima Tavallaie,Amir Ali Rahsepar, Seyyed Mohammad Reza Parizadeh, Mohammad Safariyan, Mohsen Nemati, MaryamMohammadi, Parisa Abbasi-Parizad,Sara Darbandi, Saeed Akhlaghi,and Gordon A. A. Ferns. The Effects of Body Acupuncture on Obesity, Anthropometric Parameters, Lipid Profile, and Inflammatory and ImmunologicMarkers, The ScientificWorld Journal 2012; Article ID 603539, 11 pages

91.   Ying Sun and Jiande Chen. Intestinal Electric Stimulation Decreases Fat Absorption in Rats:Therapeutic Potential for Obesity, Obes Res. 2004; 12(8): 1235–1242

92.   Katsuhiko Kohara, Masayuki Ochi, Yasuharu Tabara, Tokihisa Nagai, Michiya Igase, Tetsuro Miki. Leptin in Sarcopenic Visceral Obesity: Possible Link between Adipocytes and Myocytes, PLoS ONE, 2011; Vol. 6 Issue 9, e24633

93.   Lili Wang. Acupuncture and Cupping therapy Thigh Obese 50 cases of analysis, Chinese Journal Misdiagn, 2008; Vol. 8, 28

94.   A D Woolf, F C Breedveld, T K Kvien. Controlling the obesity epidemic is important for maintaining musculoskeletal health, Ann Rheum Dis 2006; 65:1401–1402

95.   Ruth S.M. Chan and Jean Woo. Prevention of Overweight and Obesity: How Effective is the Current Public Health Approach, Int. J. Environ. Res. Public Health 2010; 7, 765-783

96.   Xian-juan Kong, Lei Gao, Hao Peng, Xian Shi. Effects of electro-acupuncture on expression of obestatin in hypothalamus of rats with simple obesity, Journal of Chinese Integrative Medicine, 2010; Vol. 8, 5, 480-485

97.   Kotha Subbaramaiah, Louise R. Howe, Priya Bhardwaj, Baoheng Du, Claudia Gravaghi, Rhonda K. Yantiss, Xi Kathy Zhou, Victoria A. Blaho, Timothy Hla, Peiying Yang, Levy Kopelovich, Clifford A Hudis, and Andrew J. Dannenberg. Obesity is associated with inflammation and elevated aromatase expression in the mouse mammary gland, Cancer Prev Res (Phila), 2011; 4(3):329-346

98.   Nathalie M A van Emmerik, Carry M Renders, Marije van de Veer, et al. High Cardiovascular risk in severely obese young children and adolescents, Arch Dis Child 2012; 97: pages 818-821

99.   S-H Cho, J-S Lee, L Thabane, J Lee. Acupuncture for obesity: a systematic review and meta-analysis, International Journal of Obesity 2009; 33, 183–196

100.   Bonnie J. Brehm, David A. D'Alessio. Environmental Factors Influencing Obesity, Endotext.com, 2010; chapter 7

101.   C-F Liu. Electro-acupuncture as an adjunct treatment for obesity, Royal Pharmaceutical Society of Great Britain, 2010; Vol. 15, 128–129

102.   Engin Can (Enqin Zhang). Obesity, www.suntenglobal.com, 2012

103.   S-H Cho, J-S Lee, L Thabane and J Lee. Acupuncture for Obesity: a systematic review and meta-analysis, International Journal of Obesity, 2009; 33, 183-196

104.   W.P.T.James The Epidemiology of Obesity: the Size of the Problem, Blackwell

Publishing Ltd., Journal of Internal Medicine, 2008; 263: 336-352

105.   Tyehao   Lu.   TCM   and   Weight Management,   Acupuncture   Today, www.acupuncturetoday.com, 2010

106.   Osama   Hamdy,   George   T   Griffing. Obesity, www.emedicine.medcape.com/article/123702-overview, 2012

107.   Richard L. Atkinson. Etiologies of Obesity, The Management of Eating Disorders and Obesity, 2005; 105-118

108.   Gao Jian-zhi, Hou Hui-fang, LI Yan, et al. Effect of acupuncture on Lipid Metabolism in Simple Obese Rat, Journal of Xinxiang Medical College 5, 2006; 005

109.   Nicolas Stettler, Theo M. Signer and Paolo M. Suter. Electronic Games and Environmental Factors associated with Childhood Obesity in Switzerland, Obesity Research, 2004; Vol.12, 6

110.   Li Yanshuang, Li Xiaogeng. Acupuncture combined with Cupping for treatment of 52 cases of Simple Obesity, Harbin Medical Journal 3, 2011; 041

111.   P Kopelman. Health Risks associated with Overweight and Obesity, Obesity Review, 2007; 8 (suppl.1) 13-17

112.   Aviva Must, Jennifer Spadano, Eugenie H. Coakley, Alison E.Field, Graham Colditz, William H. Dietz. The Disease Burden Associated with Overweight and Obesity, JAMA, 1999; Vol. 282, No.16

113.   Aus Tariq Ali, Nigel John Crowther. Health Risks associated with Obesity, JEMDSA, 2005; Vol. 10, No.2

116.   Edward D Mun, George L. Blackburn, and Jeffrey B. Matthews. Current Status of Medical and Surgical Therapy for Obesity, Gastroenterology, 2001; 0120: 669-681

117.   Kunio Yamanouchi, Takashi Shinozaki, Kiwami Chikada, Toshihiko Nishikawa, Katsunori Ito, Shoji Shimizu. Daily Walking combined with Diet therapy is a useful means for Obese NIDDM patients Not only to reduce body weight but also to improve insulin sensitivity, Diabetes Care, 1995; Vol. 18, 6

119.   K.R. Fox and M. Hillsdon. Physical Activity and Obesity, Obesity Reviews, 2007; 8 (suppl. 1), 115-121

121. Lori M. Dickerson, Pharm D., and Peter J. Carek. Drug Therapy for Obesity, Am Fam Physician, 2000; 61 (7): 2131-2138

122. George A Bray, F Xavier Pi-Sunyer, Jean E Mulder. Drug Therapy of Obesity, UpToDate, 2010; 18.1

123. Louis J. Aronne. Drug Therapy for Obesity – A therapeutic Option? The Journal of Clinical Endocrinology & Metabolism, 1999; Vol. 84, no.1, 7-10

124. Mayo clinic staff, www.mayoclinic.com, 2012

125. Chen F, Wu S, Zhang Y, Zhen ci yan jju. Effect of Acupoint Catgut Embedding on TNF-alpha and Insulin resistance in Simple Obesity patients, Acupuncture Research, 2007; 32(1):49-52

126. Shi Y, Zhang LS, Zhao C, He CQ. Comparison of therapeutic effects of Acupuncture-Cupping plus Acupoint Catgut Embedding and Electroacupuncture on Simple Obesity of Stomach and Intestine Excess-Heat type, Chinese Acupuncture & Moxibution, 2006; 26(8): 547-50

127. Hsieh CH, Su TJ, Fang YW, Chou PH. Efficasy of two different materials used in Auricular

Acupressure on weight reduction and Abdominal Obesity, Am J Chin Med., 2012; 40(4):713-20

128.   Bu TW, Tian XL, Wang SJ, Liu W, Li XL, Tan YH. Comparison and analysis of therapeutic effects of different therapies on Simple Obesity, Zhongguo Zhen Jiu (abstrack), 2007; 27(5): 337-40

129.   Richards D, Marley J. Stimulation of Auricular Acupuncture Points in Weight Loss, Aust. Fam Physician, 1998; suppl. 2: S73-7

130.   Ai Bing-wei and Wang Qi-cai. A Clinical Series, Acupuncture and Moxibustion for Obesity, 2010; People's Medical Publishing House, Beijing, China

131.   Shi Y, Zhang LS, Zhao C, Zuo XY. Controlled study of needle warming therapy and Electroacupuncture on Simple Obesity of Spleen deficiency type, Chinese Acupuncture & Moxibution, 2005; 465

132.   Mehmet Tugrul Cabioglu, Neyhan Ergene. Changes in Levels of Serum Insulin, C-Peptide and Glucose after Electroacupuncture and Diet Therapy in Obese Women, The American Journal of Chinese Medicine, 2006; Vol. 34, No.3, 367-376

133.   Liu Zhicheng, Sun Fengmin, Z. Miaohua. Effect of Acupuncture on the Amygdala of Obese Rats, Acupuncture Research, 2000; 25.1. 18-22

134.   Xu Ming. Obesity and Physical Exercises, Journal of Chengdu Physical Education Institute 5, 2002;025

135.   Zhao Mei, Yuan Jinhong, Li Jia et al. Effect of Acupuncture on Feeding Center of Hypothalamus in Experimental Fat Rats, Chinese Acupuncture & Moxibustion 5, 2001;036

136.   Liu Zhicheng, Sun Fengmin, Han Yan. Effect of acupuncture on level of Monoamines and activity of Adenosine Triphosphatase in Lateral Hypothalamic area of Obese rats, Chinese Journal of Integrated Traditional and Western Medicine, 2000; 20(7):521-3

137.   Zhou Yong, Zhao Xia, Zhang Yu-chao, Wang Hou-lei. Changes in posture and plasma lipids and their relativity in reducing obesity by exercise, Journal of Shaanxi Normal University (Natural Science Edition), 2006

138.   Ma Cheng & Liu Zhicheng. Regulative Effects of Electroacupuncture on Gastric Hyperfunction Induced by Electro stimulation of the

Lateral Hypothalamus area of Rabbits, Acupuncture Research 2, 1994; 011

139. Liu Zhicheng, Sun Fengmin, Su Jing et al. Action of Acupuncture on Ventromedial Neucleus of Hypothalamus in the Rat of Obesity, Journal of Traditional Chinese Medicine 1, 2000; 021

140. Wei Qunli & Liu Zhicheng. Comparison between Auricular Acupuncture and Combination of Auricular and Body Acupuncture in Treating Simple Obesity, Journal of Nanjing TCM University (Natural Science), 2002; Vol. 18, 1

141. Chen Zhen Yan, Zhang Tang, Liu Yi-cheng. Electro-acupuncture plus auricular acupressure treatment in Simple Obesity Efficasy, Acupuncture Clinical Journal 2008; Vol. 24. 1

142. Liu Zhicheng et al. The Experimental Study on acupuncture Treatment of Simple Obesity in Rats, Acupuncture Research 1, 1998; 023

143. Liu Zhi-cheng, Sun Feng-min, Sun Zhi, Zhang Zhong Zhong-cheng, Zhu Miao-hua, Wei Qunli, Hong Cheng-yun. Effect of acupuncture on contents of leptin and insulin in obese rats, Modern Journal of Intergrated Traditional Chinese and Western Medicine, 2003; 006

144.   Yuji Matsuzawa, Ichiro Shimomura, Tadashi Nakamura, Yoshiaki Keno, Katsuto Tokunaga. Pathophysiology and pathogenesis of Visceral Fat Obesity, Diabetes Research and Clinical Practice, 1994; Vol 24, supplement, pages 111-116

145.   Liu Zhi-cheng, Sun Feng-min, Zhao Mei, Sun Zhi, Xiang Xiao-ren, Zhu Miao-hua, Zhang Zhong-cheng, Hong Cheng-Yun. Study of Acupuncture on arcuate nucleus of obese rats, Modern Journal of Integrated Traditional Chinese and Western Medicine, 2003; 10

146.   Zhi-cheng Liu, Feng-Min Sun, Bin Xu, Zhi Sun, Zhong-Cheng, Zhang, Bing-Guo Xu, Run-Hu Yan, Jin-Hong Yuan. Effect of acupuncture on the Neurochemical information mass in Cerebral Cortex of Obese Rats, Chinese Journal of Clinical Rehabilitation, 2004; Vol.8, 18

147.   Liu Zhi-cheng, Sun Feng-min, Wang Yi-zheng. Good Regulation of Acupuncture in Simple Obesity Patients with Stomach-Intestine Excessive Heat Type, Chinese Journal of Intergrated Traditional and Western Medicine; 1995; 3

148.   Yang Chun-zhuang, Ma Ying, Xu Yong-liang, Wang Yu, Wang Ying, Zhang Dawei. Influence of Acupuncture on Serum Leptin Level and

Hypothalamic Leptin Receptor Expression in Simple Obesity Rats, Acupuncture Research; 2007; 010

149.   Liu Zhicheng et al. The Clinical Observation on the Antiobesity effects and Lipid-reducing effects of Acupuncture and Moxibution, Chinese Journal of Rehabilitation, 1990; 03

150.   Bai Chun-yan, Zhuo Lian-shi, Zhu Yi, Fu Yan. Effect of Electroacupuncture on Hypothalamic Leptin and Leption Receptor RNA Expression in Rats with Nonalcoholic Fatty Live Disease, Acupuncture Reseach 4, 2010; 011

151.   Liu Zhichen, Sun Feng-min, Zhao Dong-hong, Zhang Zhong-cheng, Sun Zhi, Wu Hai-tao Xu Bing-guo, Zhu Miao-hua, and Li Chao-jun. Effect of Acupuncture on Uncoupling Protein 1 Gene Expression for Brown Adipose Tissue of Obese Rats, Chinese Journal of Integrated Traditional and Western Medicine, 2003; 204-209

152.   Cheng Ling, Chen Miao-gen, Yang Hui, He Jin-sen, Zhang Chun-yan, Xiao Chun-yi. Influence of Acupuncture on Insulin Resistance in Simple Obesity Patients, Shanghai Journal of Acupuncture and Moxibution, 2007; 2, R246

153.   Philip James. Obesity Surgery, 2003; 13, 329-330

154.   Ching Hsiu Hsieh, Tsann-Jnn Su, Yu-Wen Fang, Pei-Hsuan Chou. Effects of Auricular Acupressure on Weight Redection and Abdominal Obesity in Asian Yong Adults, Am. J. Chinese Medicine, 2011; 39, 433

155.   AI Bing-wei, Jiao Lin, Wang Gui-ying. Clinical Observation on Photoelectric Treatment Instrument combined with acupuncture for treatment of Simple Obesity, Chinese Acupuncture & Moxibution 10, 2006; 009

156.   Peter Deadman, Mazin Al-Khafaji, Kevin Baker, A Manual of Acupuncture, Journal of Chinese Medicine Publications, 2001; ISBN 0951054678

157.   Xiao   Zhong. www.tcmdiscovery.com/TCM-Literature, 2012

158.   Shang   Xiao-li,   Shang   Xiao-ling. Treatment of 60 cases of Simple Obesity by Acupuncture plus Tuina therapy, Journal of Acupuncture and Tuina Science, 2003; Vol. 1, 3, 42-44

159.   Li Li-qiu, Gong Wei-Zhi, Deng Xin. Treatment of Simple Obesity of Stomach-Intestine Excessive Heat Type by Acupuncture and Tuina, Journal of Acupuncture and Tuina Science, 2005; Vol. 3, 2, 61-62

160.   Xia Bo, Dr. Guan Zun-hui's Clinical Experience in treating Simple Obesity by acupuncture, Journal of Acupuncture and Tuina Science, 2003; Vol. 1, 6, 6-8

161.   Shen Tao. Treatment of Obesity with Hyperlipidemia by Cap-shaped Warm acupuncture, 2005; Vol. 3, 1, 16-17

162.   Xu Bin and Liu Zhi-cheng. Chinese-English Edition of Acupuncture for Weight Loss, Shanghai Scientific and Technical Publishers, ISBN 978-7-5323-8994-0

163.   Wang SJ, Xu HZ, Xiao HL. Effect of high frequency Electroacupuncture on Lipid Metabolism in Obesity Rats, Acupuncture Research, 2008; 33, 3, 154-158